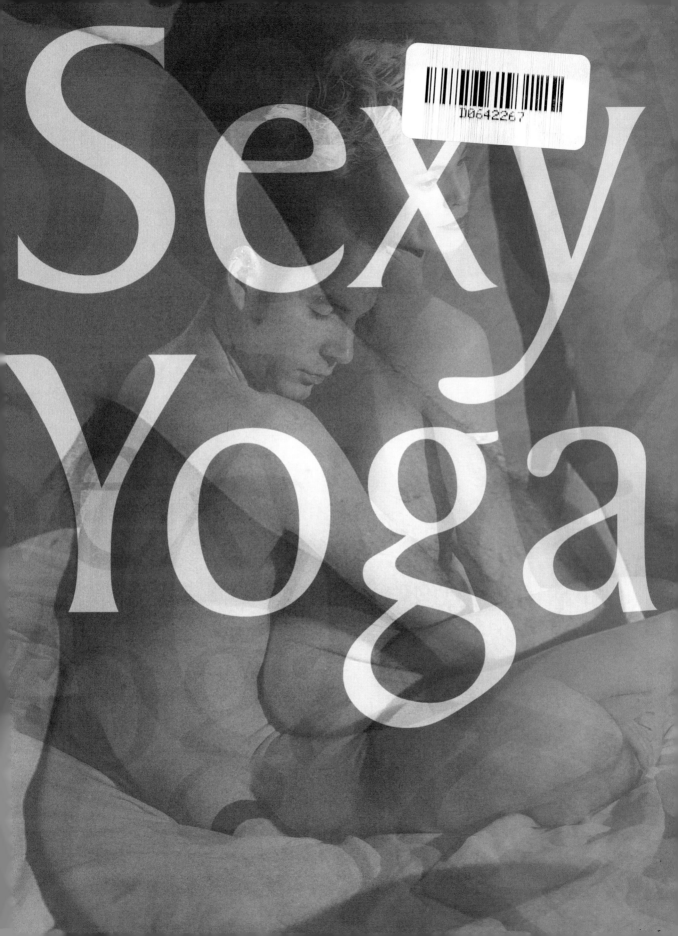

Sexy Yoga

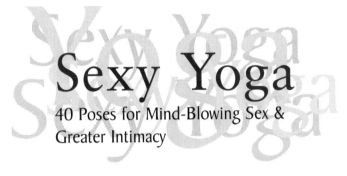

Sexy Yoga

40 Poses for Mind-Blowing Sex & Greater Intimacy

Ellen Barrett

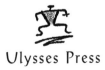

Ulysses Press

Published by: Ulysses Press
          P.O. Box 3440
          Berkeley, CA 94703
          www.ulyssespress.com

Library of Congress Control Number: 2004108865
ISBN 1-56975-436-5

Printed in Canada by Transcontinental Printing

10 9 8 7 6 5 4 3 2 1

Editorial and production staff: Ashley Chase, Lynette Ubois,
     Steven Schwartz, Claire Chun, Lily Chou
Design: Robles-Aragón
Photography: Andy Mogg
Models: Ellen Barrett, Sonya Smith, Nol Simonse

Distributed in the United States by Publishers Group West
and in Canada by Raincoast Books

This book has been written and published strictly for informational purposes, and in no way should it be used as a substitute for consultation with a health care professional. You should not consider educational material herein to be the practice of medicine or to replace consultation with a physician or other medical practitioner. The author and publisher are providing you with information in this work so that you can have the knowledge and can choose, at your own risk, to act on that knowledge. The author and publisher also urge all readers to be aware of their health status and to consult health professionals before beginning any health program, including changes in dietary habits.

Table of Contents

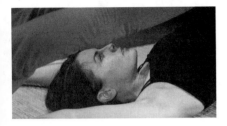

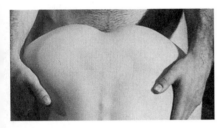

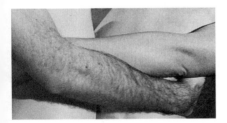

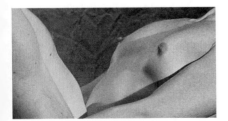

Introduction

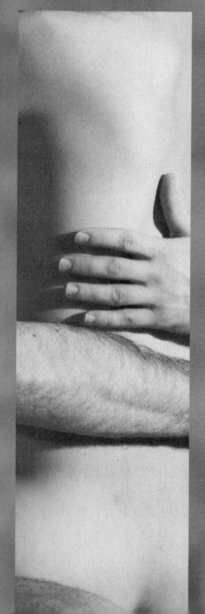

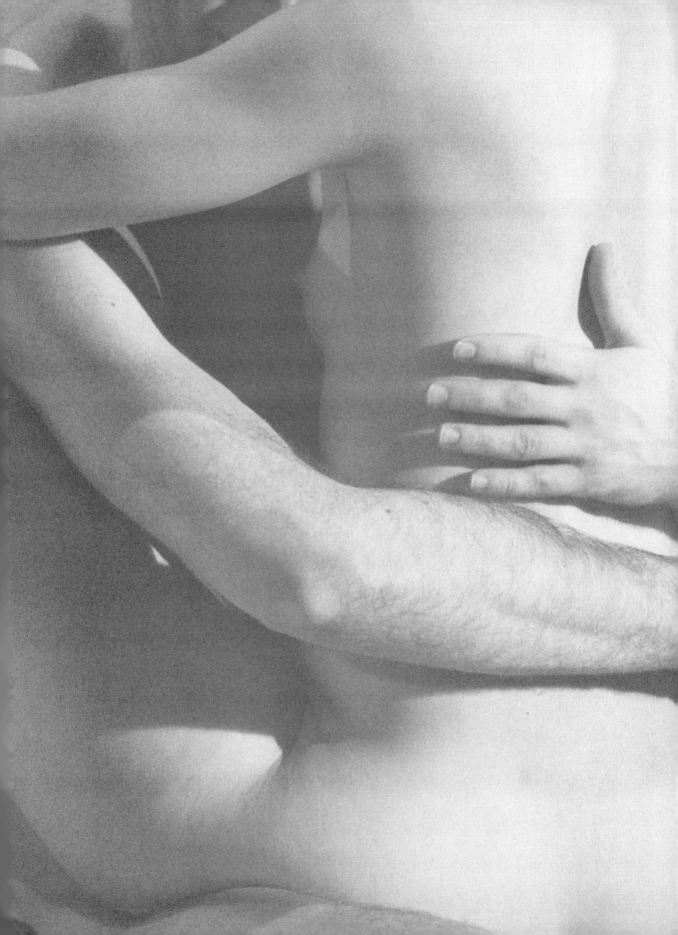

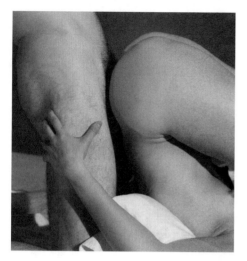

■ The Bible of Sex

THE KAMA SUTRA (A.K.A. "THE BIBLE OF SEX") is the most famous work on sex ever written. It was penned over 2000 years ago by Vatsyayana, a Hindu scholar, as a religious duty. Vatsyayana created the Kama Sutra by compiling the sexual practices documented from earlier centuries, elaborating on them with intimate detail, and then drawing explicit conclusions. The goal was to prevent divorce—for the essence of the Kama Sutra is a love manual, guiding couples toward happiness and pleasure. "Pleasures," said Vatsyayana, "are as necessary for the well-being of the body as food." Only about 20 percent of the total text is devoted to sexual positions. The remainder gives guidance on how to be a good citizen and insights into men and women in relationships, much like the popular *Men Are from Mars, Women Are from Venus*.

The Kama Sutra was composed in Sanskrit, the literary language of ancient India. In Sanskrit, *kama* means "desire" and *sutra* means "rules." So "Kama Sutra" translates as "The Rules of Desire." In 1883 Sir Richard Burton brought an English translation to the Western world—it became famous during the Victorian period, where it was labeled "erotica" and secretly circulated among wealthy Europeans and sophisticated Americans. Ironically, in that supposedly reserved time period when sexuality was denounced and repressed, the Kama Sutra was much in demand.

The Kama Sutra presents sex as sacred—essential to life, a gift from God, worthy of serious study. Even if you have never actually seen the Kama Sutra firsthand, you probably know about its 100-plus sexual positions that are graphically illustrated and analyzed. It has withstood the test of time—perhaps because of its in-depth content, or maybe because of society's insatiable hunger for better sex.

■ Modern Yoga

YOGA MEANS "UNION" IN SANSKRIT. IT WAS developed in India over 5000 years ago to promote the "union" of the mind, body and spirit. Today, yoga is mostly practiced as an exercise system that consists of a series of physical poses that bring flexibility, strength, vitality, heightened awareness and peace of mind to the practitioner. Most of the yoga forms that have found their way into the Western world, and the specific type of yoga showcased in this book, are varieties of hatha yoga. With *ha* meaning "sun" and

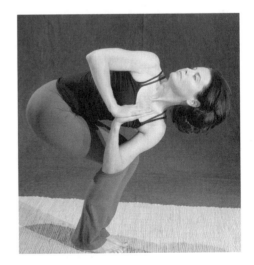

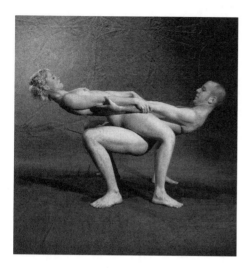

tha meaning "moon," hatha yoga is the healthy joining of opposites. It provides an excellent way for people of all ages to get in shape, develop balance and achieve a sense of centeredness.

Hatha yoga has three essential components: 1. *Asanas*, or poses; 2. *Pranayama*, or breathing control, which we discuss more deeply in a following chapter; and 3. *Pratyahara*, or meditation, which is the fundamental mind stability attained during and after practice.

■ Sex + Yoga = Sexy Yoga

BLEND THE STUDY OF THE KAMA SUTRA AND the practice of hatha yoga, and voilà—Sexy Yoga is born. Not only is it stunning how relevant the 2000-year-old love manual is in today's world—it is also fascinating how similar the sexual positions are to yoga postures.

The two disciplines possess even more common ground. For one, they both have spiritual beginnings in India. The Kama Sutra was an original Hindu religious scripture before it was translated and brought to the West as erotica literature, while yoga was thought to be an avenue toward spiritual enlightenment. Many believe it's these spiritual roots that have made the Kama

Sutra and the science of yoga withstand the test of time and obliterate cultural differences.

A second commonality it that many of the advanced sexual positions illustrated in the Kama Sutra—with their extreme flexibility and body awareness—could never be realized without a steady yoga practice. Some of the postures are awfully demanding for anyone other than an Olympic gymnast. Unless you build a strong and supple body with frequent yoga, you will find it hard to achieve the Kama Sutra poses.

The last major link between sex and yoga is that both activities have the power to cultivate acceptance and connectedness in your own body. This is a prerequisite to uniting intimately with others, as well as feeling at home in your own skin.

■ How to Use This Book

THIS BOOK IS FOR INDIVIDUALS AS WELL AS COUPLES. It's a bedside inspiration, a mindful exercise regime and a guide to more sensual sex all rolled into one. It doesn't matter if you're a yoga veteran or newcomer—we've tailored this book to meet just about everyone's needs. Of course, some of the poses may be intimidating—everyone learns his or her strengths and weaknesses. Be sure to take your time—as B.K.S Iyengar says,

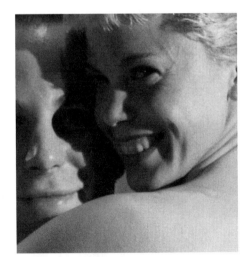

"yoga cannot be rushed," so set aside a period of time for your practice without interruption.

And, definitely, don't take this yoga too seriously. It's meant to be fun and playful, and perhaps it'll spice up your love life. Feeling inflexible? Don't get discouraged. Several of these poses require an extensive yoga background. We've included them for your visual pleasure and perhaps as something to aspire toward in the future. Listen to your body, keep breathing and do your best. In fact, just doing your best is sunshine for your soul.

We begin with Glowing Solo—a series of traditional poses that stimulate the sexual chakras, introducing your body to the deeply sensual nature of yoga. The solo poses prepare you for the Divine Duets, intimate couple yoga poses based on positions from the Kama Sutra. These same positions become ecstatic and spiritual sexual experiences in the last section, Sacred Sex.

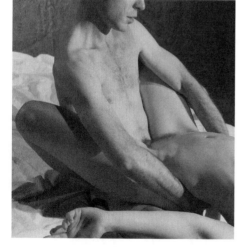

■ Safety

BE SURE TO LISTEN TO YOUR BODY'S NEEDS. You should be able to decipher the difference between "challenge" and "pain." Try to practice with your muscles warm. If you and your partner plan on being naked, be sure to turn up the thermostat to prevent muscle strain. Warm muscles have more give; colder muscles are at a higher risk for injury. If you are pregnant, consult a prenatal yoga teacher for the appropriate protocol. Avoid inverted poses if you are menstruating. Don't wear shoes or socks—you want your feet to be uninhibited. Yoga is best practiced on an empty stomach. If this is not possible, wait two to three hours after eating before practicing.

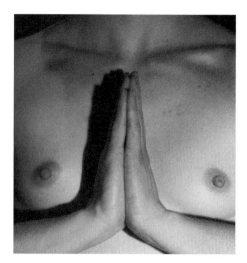

■ Breathing for Better Sex

FOR MOST OF THE DAY, BREATHING IS INVOLUNTARY and goes unnoticed. In today's Western world, we seem to talk incessantly about what (and what not) to eat and drink, and ironically breathing—being the number-one instant energy giver—goes with little attention. Yoga, however, gives breathing top billing!

Many yoga scholars believe that the act of conscious breathing *is* yoga in its purest form, while many sex therapists utilize breathing techniques as tools for better sex. Breathing is a proven energy booster, stress buster and mood enhancer—as is great sex! It makes perfect sense to intermingle breathing and sex. By fusing them together, we can magnify these much desired results.

Ujjayi, Sanskrit for "victorious uprising," is one of the most widely used breathing techniques for hatha yoga and meditation. It's slow, deliberate and calming. The technique is simple: With your mouth closed, draw in air through your nose and allow your ribs to expand sideways, filling the lungs from the bottom up. Your shoulders should remain motionless. Pause at the top of the full inhale, then exhale out through your nose or mouth. It should sound like the ocean, with the sound coming from your throat, not your nose.

Try inhaling to a count of four. Then hold your breath, counting to two, and start exhaling slowly, again to a count of four. Breathing in and out to an equal number of beats is called rhythmic breathing. You allow four beats to fill your lungs, two to retain the breath, and four to breathe out.

EXERCISE: SYNCHRONIZED BREATHING

THE UNION OF BREATH IS PERFECT FOREPLAY, SETTING A RHYTHM
FOR THINGS TO COME.

Sit cross-legged and back to back. Lean against your partner and comfortably hold hands. Using the *Ujjayi* technique explained above, begin breathing. As your partner inhales, you inhale. As they exhale, you exhale. Try to elongate each breath and also match the duration of your inhale and exhale. You can do this by counting to five on the inhale and then, at the same tempo, count to five on the exhale. You'll be able to feel your partner's ribcage expand during this activity, and you'll also notice how deeply he or she breathes. Try not to talk—let your breathing be the only form of communication for now.

There are two mental scenes to remember: 1. When inhaling, imagine a balloon filling up with helium, as if floating up to the sky. 2. When exhaling, imagine all the unwanted toxins and stress exiting your body through your nose.

Try to maintain *Ujjayi* breathing during all of the poses described in these pages. It will help your body stay warm, it will lower your risk of injury and it will keep your mind focused on the present moment. There is also something incredibly sensual about hearing and feeling the breeze of your partner's breath against your skin.

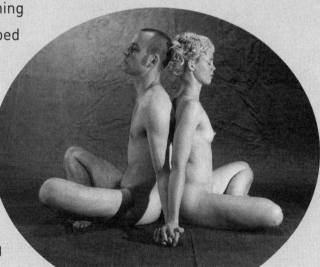

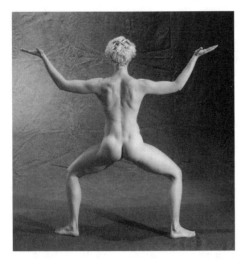

■ The Chakra System

ACCORDING TO EASTERN PHILOSOPHY, YOUR SEX life is governed by your chakras. When your chakras are in healthy working order, you'll find your sexual relations to be vibrant and healthy too. This correspondence is the reason we dedicate an entire chapter to the chakra system.

Chakras are energy whirlpools that reside in and around the human body. In Sanskrit, yoga's native language, *chakrum* translates as "wheel." There are seven main chakra energy centers, and while *Sexy Yoga* primarily focuses on the sexiest three—the root, sacral and heart chakras—all seven are of equal importance, since everything in your body is interconnected. The wheels of your chakra system must work in sync just as the wheels of a clock must work together.

The seven chakras are as follows:

The *root*—The most primitive in nature, this chakra relates to the need to survive and reproduce. It is home to all sexual organs and functions in men and some of the sexual organs and functions in women.

The *sacral*—The second chakra relates to intuition, confidence in one's self and sexual functions and emotion (in women).

The *solar plexus*—This is the center of personal power, connected to the ego. It also plays a major role in digestion.

The *heart chakra*—In the middle of the heart and the lungs, this chakra regulates breathing and circulation and is home to the center of love in the human body.

The *throat chakra*—Located on the throat, this chakra controls one's voice and one's ability to communicate.

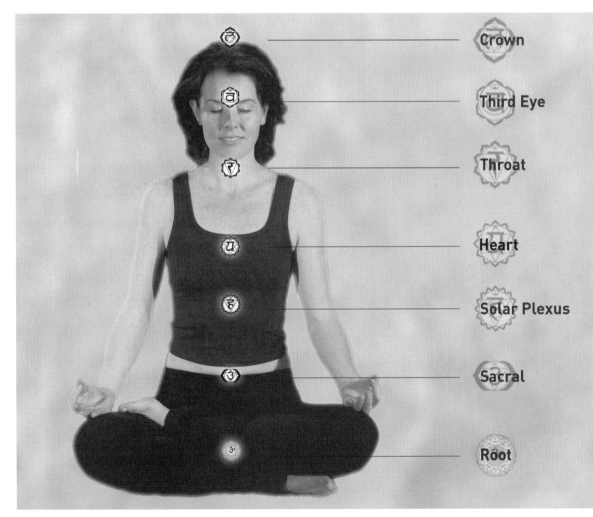

Crown

Third Eye

Throat

Heart

Solar Plexus

Sacral

Root

The *third eye*—On one's forehead, this chakra is related to vision—both physical eye health and psychic vision.

The *crown*—This chakra is related to the brain, and especially the pituitary and pineal glands. It sits above the head like a halo. It's the highest chakra, responsible for spiritual, emotional and mental enlightenment.

Since our goal in this book is to enhance our sexuality, we are most concerned with stimulating the three chakras that play direct roles in love, sex and interpersonal relations: the root, heart and sacral chakras.

■ Aura Alert

THE ENERGY FIELD AROUND EVERY HUMAN BEING is one's aura—much of the color and energy of the aura is supplied by the chakras. Have you ever been attracted to someone who you knew wasn't "your type" but for some reason you harbored strong desire nonetheless? It was probably their aura that turned you on. Sexual chemistry between two people is often thought to derive from their compatible auras. You can feel the presence of someone whose aura is supplied with open, stimulated and balanced chakras. They often have a charismatic magnetism that oozes sexual vigor and vitality.

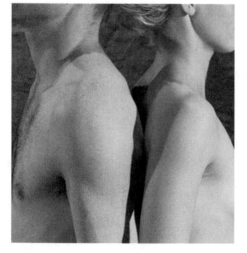

EXERCISE: SENSING YOUR PARTNER'S AURA

Sit back to back, either on pillows or directly on the floor. Position yourself about one inch away from each other. You don't want to be touching at all. Now close your eyes and bring all your attention to your spine. Feel the heat radiating between your backs and try to observe the subtlety of the heat's origin. This is a nice way to commence foreplay, since here you shut off all your attention to outside stimuli other than your partner.

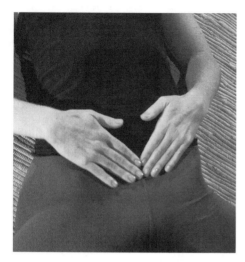

■ Sex, Yoga and the Chakras

WHERE DOES YOGA FIT IN WITH SEX AND THE chakras? For one, yoga is sensual, spiritual and sexual. Second, many of the yoga postures you see in this book have been developed to keep the chakra system—and the natural harmony within the human body—balanced. A good yoga instructor will often direct students to their own chakras in hopes of higher awareness. Third, the chakra system, yoga and the original Kama Sutra text are siblings, born from Mother India. Triplets, indeed!

We all know that yoga is great exercise and it's wonderful for overall health. What I want to express in the pages of *Sexy Yoga* is that yoga is also monumentally helpful when it comes to sex. In this day and age, we tend to seek out pills, potions and other external things to "fix" or improve our sexual inadequacies. Maybe you are not enjoying sex as much as you once did or perhaps your libido seems low. Well, the "cure" is within you already and can be explored in yoga poses. Yoga, especially the postures contained within these pages, can be your highway to sensational sex.

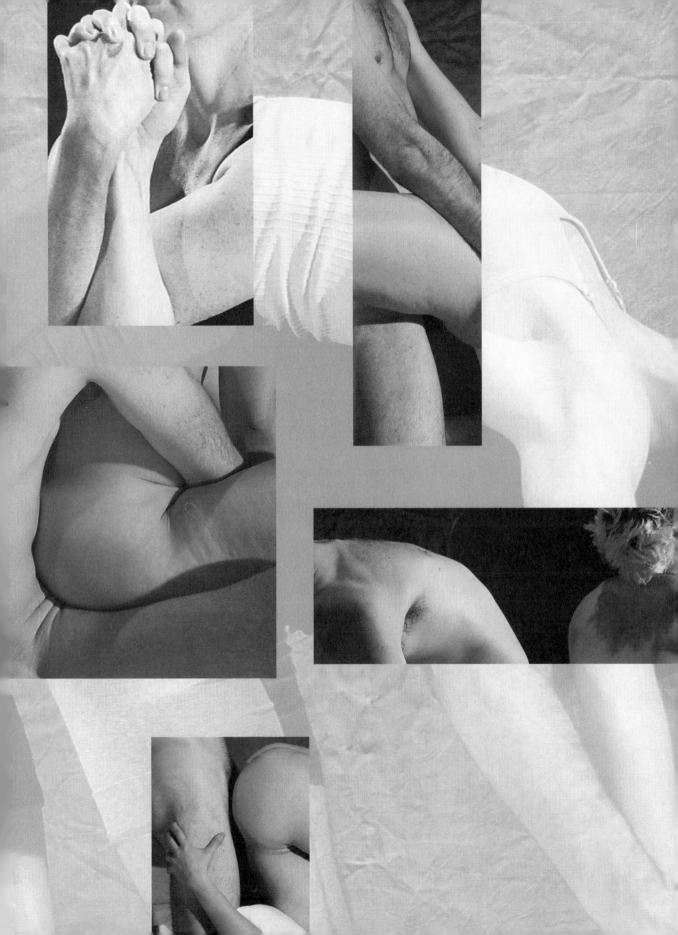

Glowing Solo

You don't need a partner to practice sexy yoga. You just need a little time and a small space. Here you will get in touch with yourself and your body, and you'll experience the loveliness you already possess.

The poses of this section produce three very rewarding results for both men and women. First, they cleanse and tone the sexual organs. This keeps us healthy and vital—enhancing our endurance in the bedroom. Second, they stimulate the three chakras (root, sacral and heart) that correlate most significantly to sex. I call this the "Natural Viagra Effect." When these chakras are opened and stimulated, your sex drive improves, as does your sexual endurance. Third, the poses prepare you for the Divine Duets and Sacred Sex sections—you'll improve agility in your hips, thighs and groin, making those exotic Kama Sutra positions much easier to manage.

The following twenty poses are listed in a specific order, and I recommend performing them in this order. The "Glowing Solo" sequence begins with standing, where you heat your deepest muscles and gently awaken your spine. It progresses to seated and kneeling poses, where more attention is placed on increasing flexibility. All of this prepares you for the third part of the sequence, the supine poses, which unlock the heart and sacral chakras, releasing euphoric feelings, better breathing and calming energy. There is always an alternative—a modification—to the main pose. If you feel a pose eluding you, try the modification instead. You'll reap many of the same benefits and stay on course.

Standing
Gentle Back Bend

Sthita Padam Bhujangasana

Setup: Stand with feet together, inner edges touching. As you inhale, raise both arms over your head, interlacing all fingers except your index fingers. Lift your torso up and off your waist and lean back. Imagine tracing the ceiling with your index fingers. The energy moves up and back while your feet remain grounded on the floor.

Duration: Hold for three to five breaths, then gently retrace your path in reverse to release.

Benefits: Opens heart and sacral chakras simultaneously, for improved circulation within the sexual organs in women and an increase in emotional well-being. One's capacity for intimacy grows in direct proportion to the openness of the heart chakra.

Modification: People commonly feel discomfort in the lower back while performing this pose. If that is the case for you, place both hands on the lower back, with fingers pointing down. This will support you as you bend your back backwards in a more conservative motion.

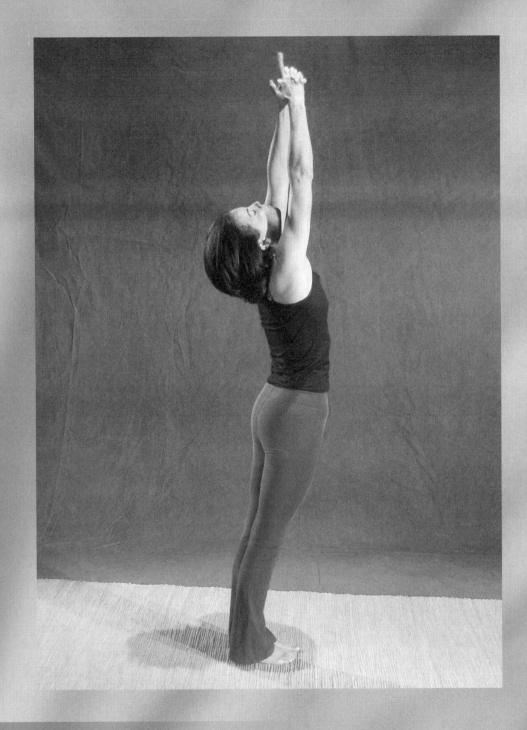

Meditation: Bring all attention to the heart. First feel its beat, then feel it expand and open as any bottled-up emotion now has an opportunity to release.

Eagle Pose

Garudasana

Setup: Stand with your feet together. Extend both arms overhead as you inhale, then exhale, bring arms halfway down and swing the right arm under the left. Cross and twist the arms like ropes. Your palms should match up. Next, bend your knees, pick up the right leg, cross it over your left and tuck your right foot behind your left ankle. Keep pulling the elbows down toward your navel and keep bending the standing knee.

Duration: Hold for five full breaths, then repeat on the other side.

Benefits: Eagle Pose is known for its thorough cleansing of the sexual organs. It produces a tourniquet effect with the root chakra. We squeeze our legs together so tightly that we temporarily block the flow of blood. So, when we release from the pose, a strong "push" of fresh oxygenated blood travels in and around the root chakra, providing an amazing cleansing benefit. With the toxins and excess stress removed from the root chakra, the vagina is much more responsive to touch and the penis functions optimally.

Modification: If balance is difficult, just cross your legs and keep your arms out like airplane wings. Your arms will assist in finding equilibrium.

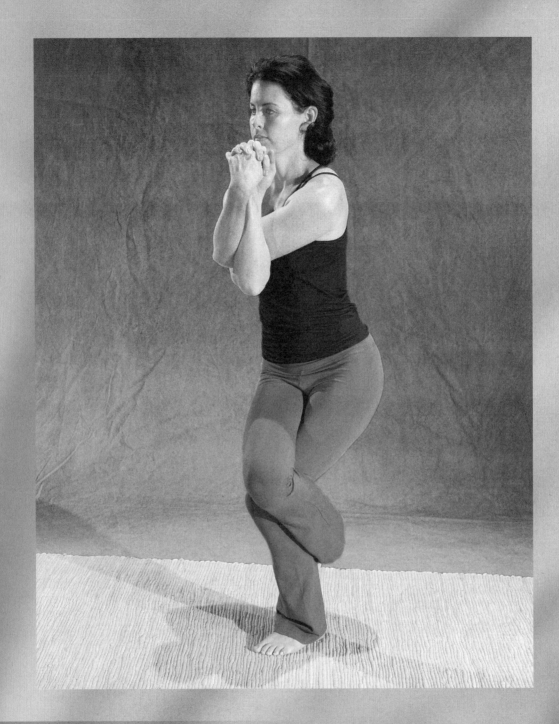

Meditation: Eagle Pose takes balance, so fix your gaze and breathe into your sacral chakra. Your thoughts and your energies are both swirling around your lower abdomen.

Prayer Twist

Namaskar Utkatasana

Setup: Stand with the inside edges of your feet touching, bend your knees and squat as if you were sitting in a chair. Bring your hands into prayer, then exhale and twist your body to face the left. Try to press your left arm outside the right thigh. On the next exhale, twist deeper and press both thumbs in towards your breast bone. Gazing upwards, over your right shoulder, is the final step.

Duration: Hold for 30 to 60 seconds, then repeat twisting while twisting to the right.

Benefits: This pose brings energy to the root chakra and stimulates circulation, while cleansing the sacral chakra region of excess tension. Plus, Prayer Twist heats up the leg muscles for increased safety in the postures to come.

Modification: If you are having difficulty twisting, try bending your knees less.

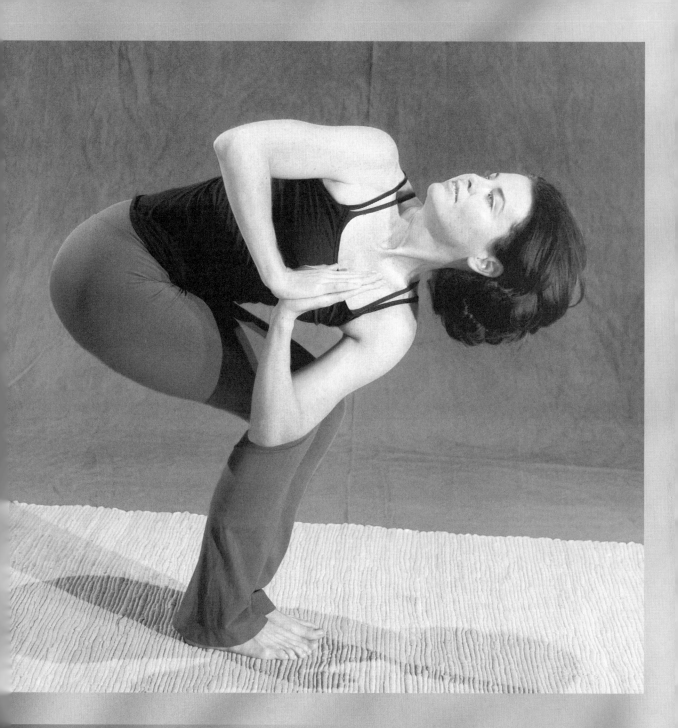

Meditation: Bring all of your attention to your pelvic floor, especially your root chakra. Softly breathe *prana* into that area and imagine energy flowing smoothly throughout this sexual region.

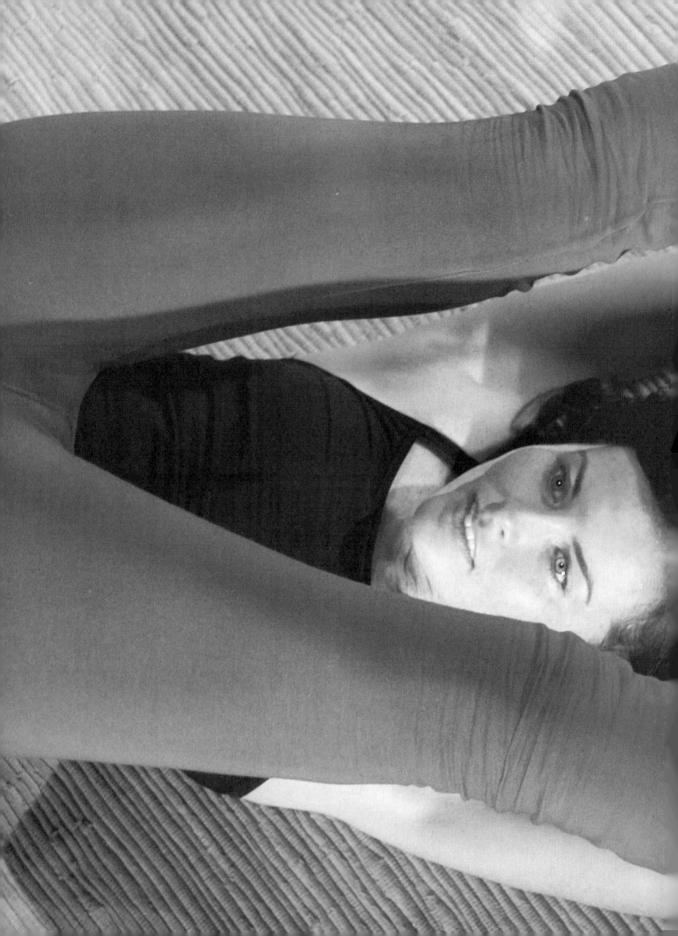

Prana

Prana is the Sanskrit word meaning "life energy." Yoga is thought to increase the flow of *prana* throughout the entire body due to its emphasis on breathing, spiritual communion and deep movement.

Spread Leg Forward Bend

Prasarita Padottanasana

Setup: Stand with your feet apart anywhere from 3 to 4½ feet (depending on your height: taller people should step wider). Rest your hands on your hips. Make sure the inner sides of your feet are parallel to each other. Engage the thigh muscles by drawing them up. Exhale and, maintaining the length of the front of your torso, lean your torso forward from the hip joints. As your torso approaches parallel to the floor, press your fingertips onto the floor directly below your shoulders. Push the top of your thighs straight back to help lengthen the front of your torso and draw the inner groins away from each other to widen the base of your pelvis. If possible, rest the crown of your head on the floor.

Benefits: Prepares the hips, thighs and groins for the Divine Duet poses.

Duration: Stay in the pose anywhere from 30 seconds to 1 minute. To come out, inhale, rest your hands on your hips, pull your tail bone down toward the floor, and swing the torso up.

Modification: Feel free to keep a slight bend in both knees if this pose feels too demanding on the lower back or hamstrings area.

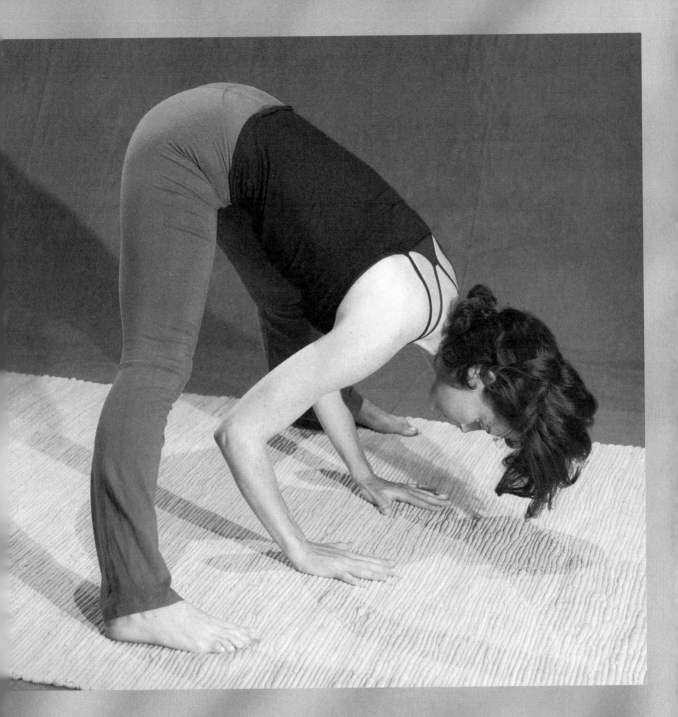

Meditation: Bring all of your attention to your pelvic floor, especially your root chakra. Softly breathe *prana* into that area and imagine energy flowing smoothly throughout this sexual region.

Frog Pose

Bhekasana

Setup: Start in the Spread Leg Forward Bend Pose (see page 32) and walk your hands away from your body until your belly touches the floor, then prop your upper body up with your forearms with your hands in a prayer position. Maintain the wide stance during the entire pose. The insides of both feet, as well as the insides of both knees, are pressing against the ground. Gently attempt to bring the hips as close to the floor as possible.

Duration: Hold for ten full breaths, then mindfully push up to your hands and walk back to forward bend.

Benefits: This posture is a perfect warmup for many of the Divine Duets. You really challenge your hip and groin muscles, which makes this pose a great way to prepare for the more advanced sexual positions.

Modification: If your knees hurt during this pose, use a blanket or towel underneath your knees as padding.

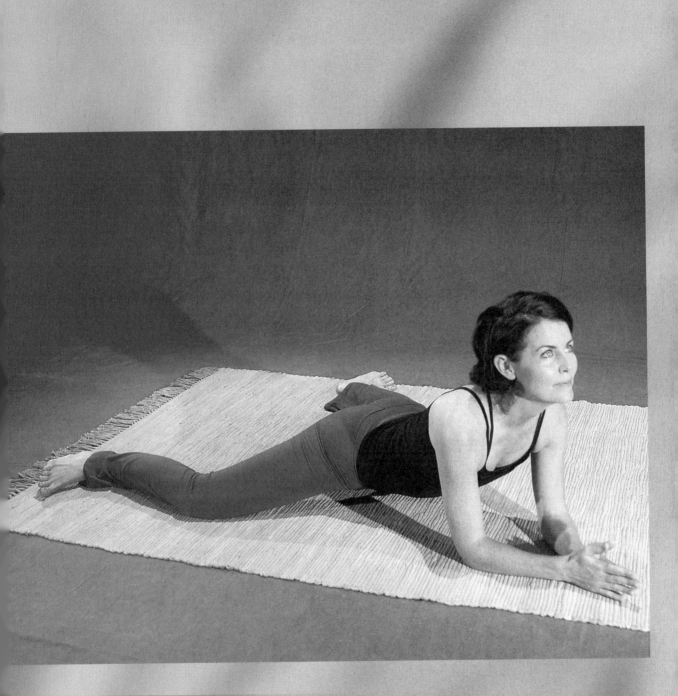

Meditation: Bring all of your attention to your pelvic floor, especially your root chakra. Softly breathe *prana* into that area and imagine energy flowing smoothly throughout this sexual region.

Crane Pose

Bakasana

Setup: Squat down with the inner sides of your feet a few inches apart. Separate your knees wider than your hips and lean your torso forward. Stretch your arms forward, then bend your elbows, place your hands on the floor and the backs of your upper arms against your shins. Snuggle your inner thighs against the sides of your torso and your shins into your armpits. Slide your upper arms down as low onto your shins as possible. Lift up onto the balls of your feet and lean forward even more, taking the weight of your torso onto the backs of your upper arms. In *Bakasana* you consciously attempt to contract your front torso and round your back completely. The inner knees should be glued to the outer arms, high up near the armpits. Keep your head in a neutral position with your eyes looking at the floor.

Duration: Stay in the pose anywhere from 20 seconds to 1 minute.

Benefits: This is a nice stimulant for the root chakra, relaxing the sexual organs in men, relaxing the vagina wall in women. At the same time it improves flexibility in the groin. You'll gain incredible abdominal strength too.

Modification: When first learning this pose, you might want to stop at the moment just before the feet lift off the ground. To release, exhale and slowly lower your feet to the floor, back into a squat.

Meditation: Bring your attention to your breath and let it swirl around your lower abdomen into your root chakra.

Reverse Crane
or "Firefly" Pose

Tittibhasana

Setup: Stand with your feet two inches wider than hip distance apart. Reach down and touch the floor with both hands inside the ankles. Bend both knees and drop your hips—you'll feel the weight shift from your feet into your hands. Your inner thighs should be hugging your upper arms. Balance on your hands and cross your ankles.

Duration: Ideally, hold for five full breaths, then uncross your ankles to release.

Benefits: This is a nice stimulant for the root chakra, while at the same time improving flexibility in the groin. You'll gain incredible abdominal strength too.

Modification: This is a very challenging pose initially, so work on getting your palms flat to the floor, and don't attempt to lift your feet up until you feel you are ready.

Meditation: Bring your attention to your breath and let it swirl around your lower abdomen into your root chakra.

Triangle

Trikonasana

Setup: Stand with your feet approximately four feet wide and your arms reaching in opposite directions. Turn your right foot to 90 degrees and pivot your left foot slightly to the right. With two straight knees and two straight arms, tilt your body to the right until your right hand rests on your lower shin. Look up toward your left thumb and continue to reach your arms in opposition.

Duration: Hold for five full breaths, then exhale and return to standing.

Benefits: This pose is unique in that all three of the sexual chakras (the root, sacral and heart) are opened and stimulated simultaneously.

Modification: If you have tight hamstrings and/or tight lower back muscles, maintain a slight bend in the front knee.

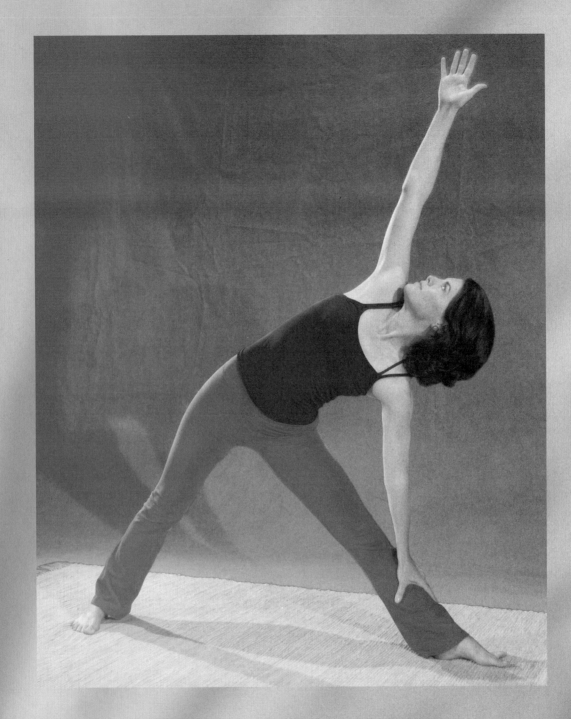

Meditation: Feel the connections between the root, sacral and heart chakras, visualizing energy surging between the three energy centers.

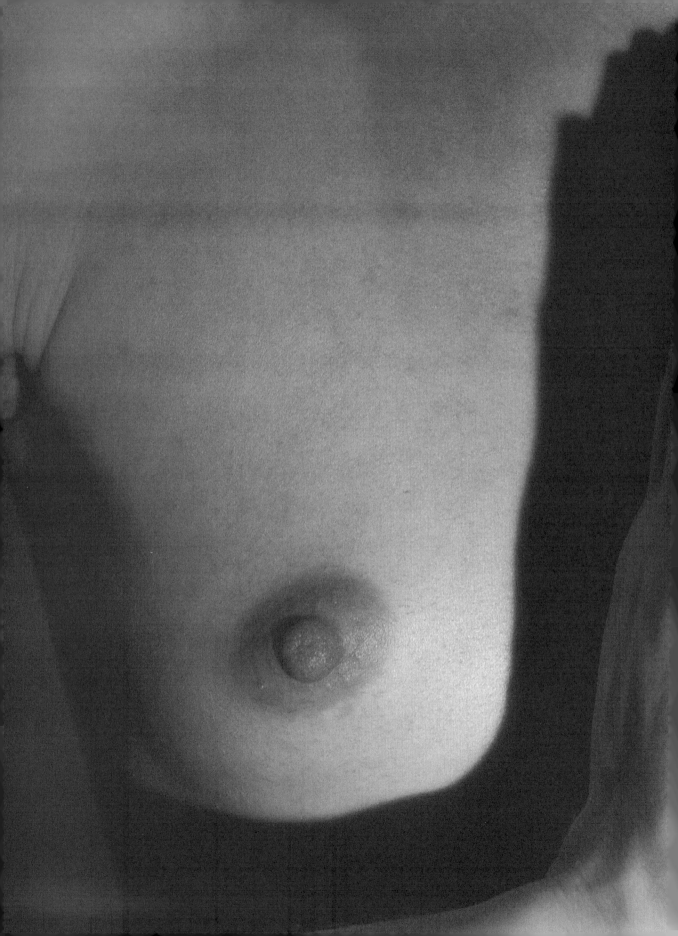

The Heart Chakra

The heart chakra is located on the same level as the physical heart, but in the center of the body. There is a marriage between the heart and the lungs—Hinduism refers to this marriage as "love and live." You can't have one without the other.

If this chakra is understimulated: Physical illnesses, including heart disease, high blood pressure and breathing troubles, result when the heart chakra is not open. Emotional diseases result as well, like lack of compassion and an inability to love one's self or others. Friendliness tends to be stifled. Physical touching produces anxiety and is often shunned.

If this chakra is open: People with openness here are warm and friendly and have high emotional intelligence. They can relate well with others sexually, and physical touch is reciprocated, rather than shunned.

Camel

Ustrasana

Setup: Kneel on the floor with your knees six to eight inches apart and your hands at your lower back. Inhale and stretch the spine up, so your ribcage feels lifted up off your waist. Exhale, and slowly release your head back, as if you're getting a shampoo. Continue bending your spine and pressing your hips forward. Place your right hand on your right heel, your left hand on your left heel. Try to keep your mouth closed and your eyes open and be sure to maintain a calm breath.

Duration: Hold for approximately 30 to 60 seconds

Benefits: Camel promotes better breathing and clearer thought, and strengthens the back. It is one of the all-time best heart chakra openers—improving intimacy with one's self and with others—and it may boost your sex drive too. If you have a hard time showing affection toward others, this posture can help you.

Modification: It's very common to experience pain in your lower back while attempting Camel. If this is the case for you, keep your hands at your lower back.

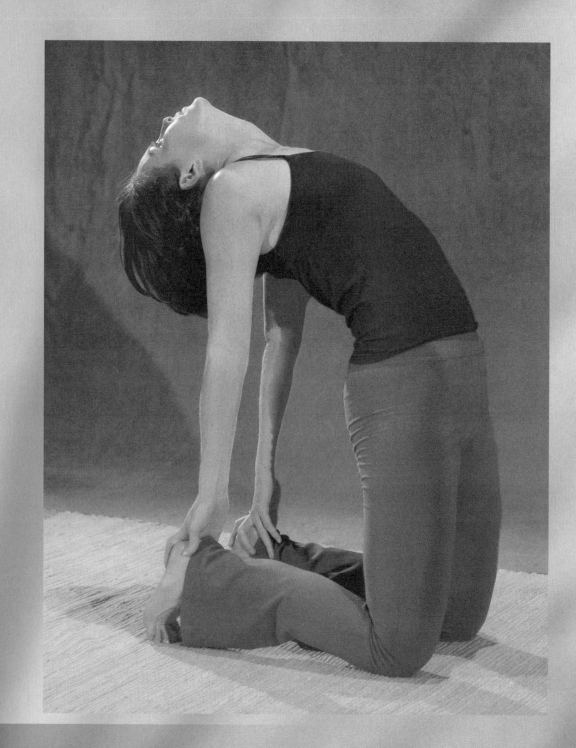

Meditation: Contemplate "love reciprocity"—the two-way flow between a healthy love of yourself and a great love for others. Feel your ability to love—to be loved and demonstrate love—grow and develop.

Forward Hero's Pose

Virasana

Setup: Sit with your butt on your heels, then slide your heels out to the side, next to your hips, so your butt releases down to touch the floor. At first, sit upright with a straight spine and settle into the posture. When ready, inhale and raise both arms up, so elbows are next to the ears, and extend your torso forward, draping the body over the knees. Keep your butt on the floor.

Duration: Hold for 10 full breaths, then exhale and release up.

Benefits: Forward Hero's Pose is especially great for women, since it regulates menstrual flow and relieves pelvic congestion. It's also great for improving knee flexibility, which is vital in many of the Divine Duets.

Modification: You may need to sit on a block or a towel if you feel discomfort in your knees. You always have the option of staying upright as well.

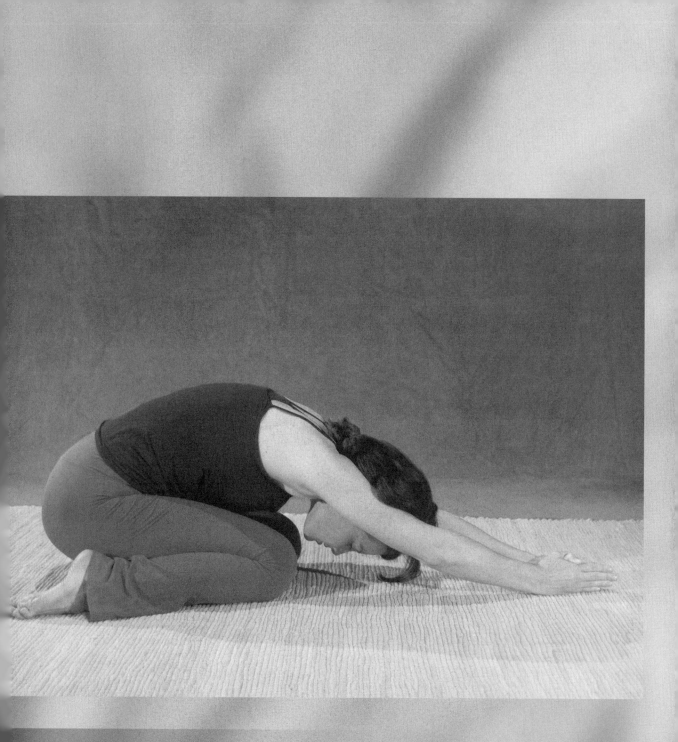

Meditation: Focus on releasing stress in the hips and groin. Your breath should sound like gentle ocean waves. Let that rhythm enter your body, bringing tranquility inside and out.

Seated Angle Pose

Baddha Konasana

Setup: Sit on the floor with the soles of your feet together. Interlock your fingers around your two big toes and straighten your spine. Try to bring your feet as close to your body as possible. Let your knees relax toward the floor and be sure to stay lifted in the chest.

Duration: Hold for 10 full breaths.

Benefits: You'll gain inner and outer thigh and knee flexibility, which will help in some of the more advanced sexual positions. This pose also opens the root chakra, which cleanses the sexual organs.

Modification: Make more of a "diamond" shape with your legs, if necessary. This will ease the discomfort in your knees.

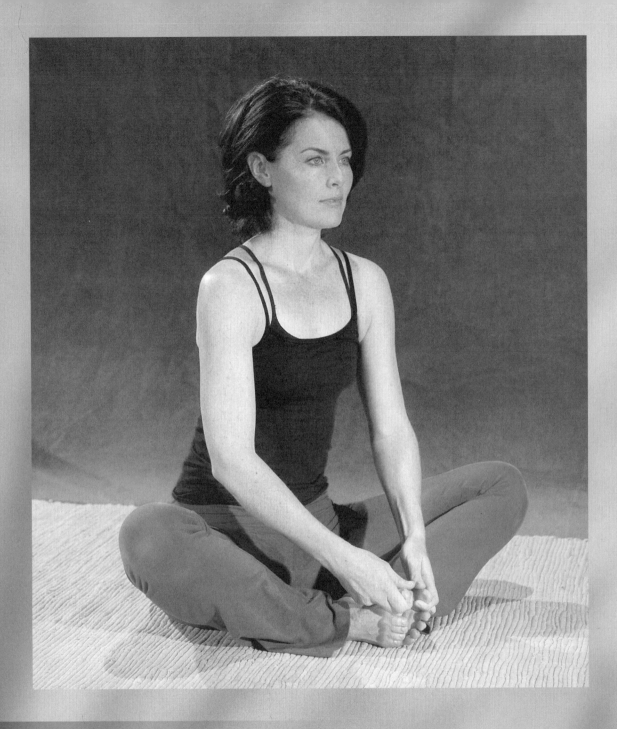

Meditation: Bring all of your attention to your pelvic floor, especially your root chakra. Softly breathe *prana* into that area and imagine energy flowing smoothly throughout this sexual region.

Seated Open Angle Pose

Upavista Konasana

Setup: Sit on the floor with your legs straddled wide apart, with your feet flexed. Squeeze your thigh muscles to "lift" your kneecaps up toward the hips. This engages the muscles of the legs, preventing muscle strain. Grasp your big toes with the first two fingers of each hand. Press your hips forward, working more deeply into the pose.

Duration: Hold for 10 full breaths.

Benefits: In this pose, you increase the flexibility in your hips, thighs and groin. You also open and stimulate the root and sacral chakras, which cleanses every sexual organ in both men and women

Modification: If flexibility in your hips is limited, you can make the stance less wide and add a slight micro-bend to the knees.

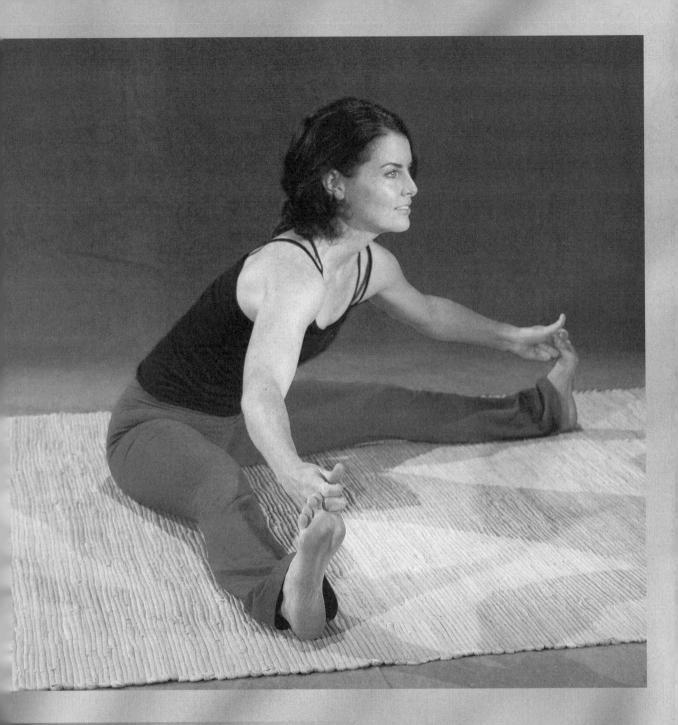

Meditation: Bring all of your attention to your pelvic floor, especially your root chakra. Softly breathe *prana* into that area and imagine energy flowing smoothly throughout this sexual region.

Bridge

Setu Bandha

Setup: Lie on your back with your arms relaxed by your sides, knees bent and feet planted hip width apart directly below the knees. On your next exhale, push your hips up off the ground. Try to lift using only your lower back, not by squeezing the buttock muscles. Also, be sure to keep your chin away from your chest. Body weight should be distributed evenly between the shoulders and the feet. Breathe deeply, stay calm and feel your spine lengthen in opposition. An optional final step is to firmly interlace your fingers, with the heels of the hands together, underneath your back.

Duration: Hold for four long, slow breathing cycles (approximately 30 seconds).

Benefits: The Bridge Pose gently heats the body, making it a great way to begin the solo series. It opens the heart center for improved intimacy with one's self and others. It aids in the release of bottled-up emotion. Some yogis believe this posture can help people recover from a broken heart.

Modification: If you are nursing a back injury or feeling too much challenge with this pose, try this: Place your hands at your lower back for extra support at the spine. This acts like a support beam.

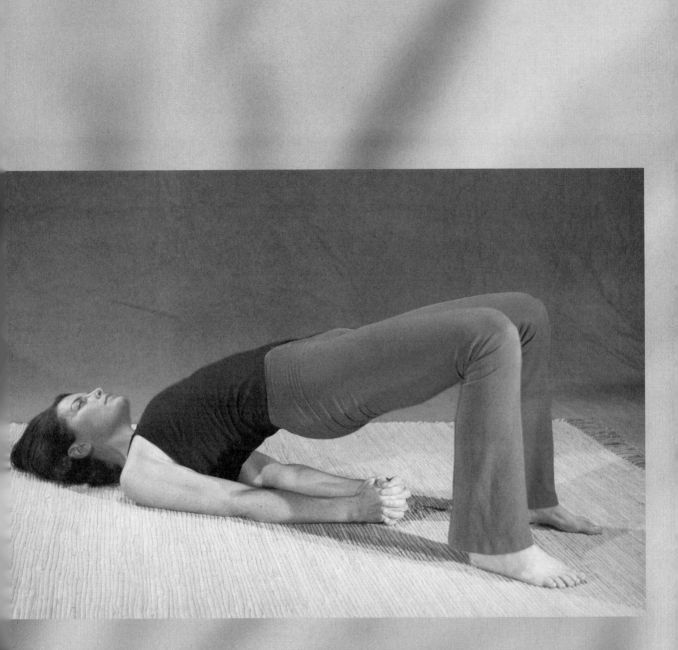

Meditation: Bring your attention to the heart. First feel its beat, then feel it expand and open as any bottled-up emotion now has an opportunity to release.

Back Bend

Urdhva Dhanurasana

Setup: Lie on your back and bend your knees, placing your heels close to your butt, hip distance apart. Place your hands under your shoulders, fingers pointing toward your feet. On an exhale, use your leg strength to lift your hips off the floor and use your arm strength to press your head and shoulders up. It feels like an inverted push-up.

Duration: Hold for five full breaths, then slowly release and rest on the floor.

Benefits: This pose provides the heart chakra with incredible stimulation, which in turn helps with the emotional side of sex. Your capacity for intimacy grows in direct proportion to the openness of your heart chakra.

Modification: The Bridge Pose is a nice alternative if you find this pose pinching your lower back.

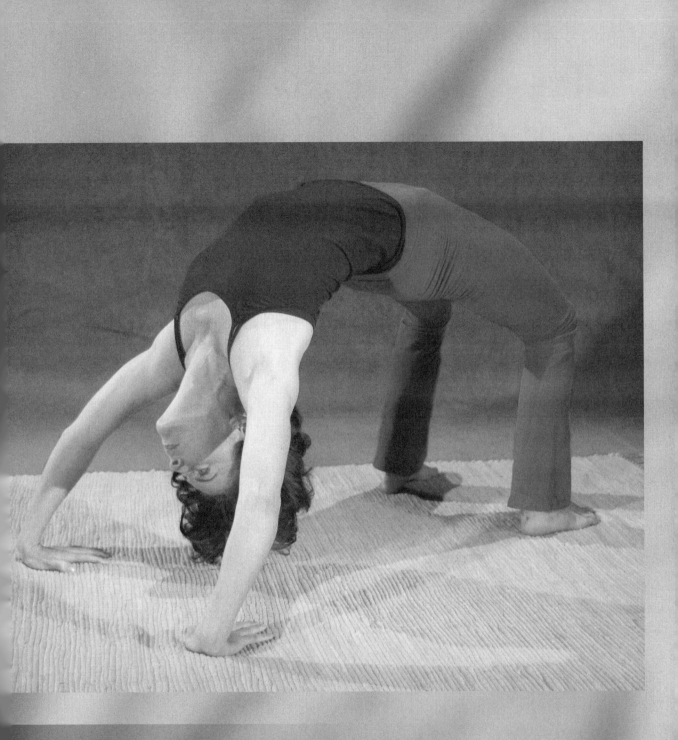

Meditation: Bring your attention to the heart. First feel its beat, then feel it expand and open as any bottled-up emotion now has an opportunity to release.

Sleeping Angle

Supta Konasana

Setup: Start on your back with your legs straight up, making a 90-degree angle. Reach up and grab your big toes with the first two fingers of each hand. Stretch your legs long, ideally until both your arms and legs are straight. Now exhale and roll up onto your shoulders, bringing your legs over your head to the floor. By keeping your chin away from your chest, you'll be sure to keep the back of your neck off the ground, which is mandatory for this pose.

Duration: Hold for five full breaths, then exhale and roll out to release.

Benefits: Sleeping Angle prepares you for the Divine Duets by stretching hip, thigh and groin muscles. This pose also opens the root chakra, which cleanses the sexual organs.

Modification: Keep your knees slightly bent if you feel tightness in the backs of your thighs.

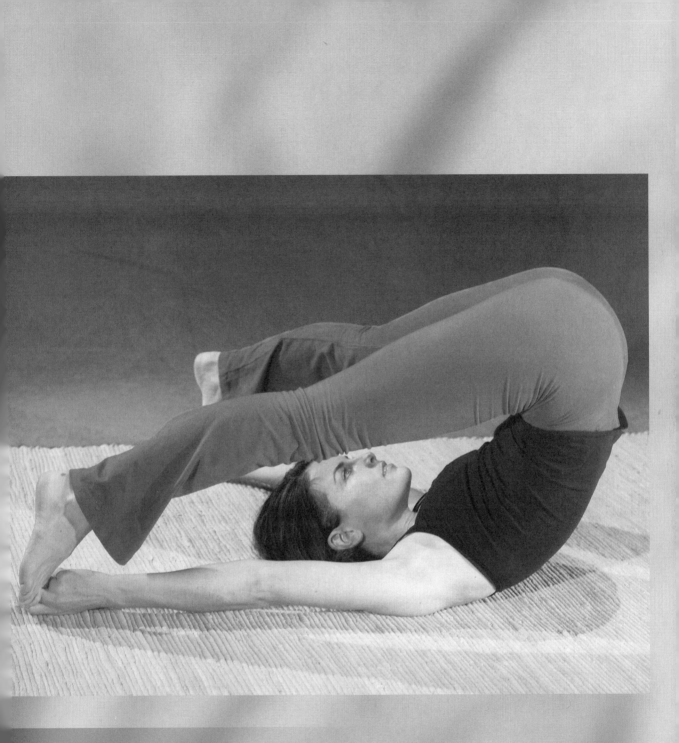

Meditation: Bring all of your attention to your pelvic floor, especially your root chakra. Softly breathe *prana* into that area and imagine energy flowing smoothly throughout this sexual region.

Plow

Halasana

Setup: Lie on your back with your arms relaxed by your sides, legs straight up—the body forms a perfect 90-degree angle. Exhale, squeeze abdominal muscles and bring both legs up and overhead. Your toes should ideally touch the floor behind your head and your knees should stay straight. Be sure to keep your chin away from your chest. Keep your abdominals pulled in and maintain an even flow of breath.

Duration: Eight full breathing cycles (approximately 60 seconds).

Benefits: Plow revitalizes the spirit. It helps you get better acquainted with the root chakra. It also improves flexibility of the spine and releases tension in the pelvis, which promotes more pleasurable sexual experiences, especially for women.

Modification: Is it difficult for you to straighten your legs fully? Then you have tight hamstrings and you should simply remain at the 90-degree angle instead of the full Plow. Over time, the hamstrings will gain more flexibility and you'll easily be able to move into the full Plow.

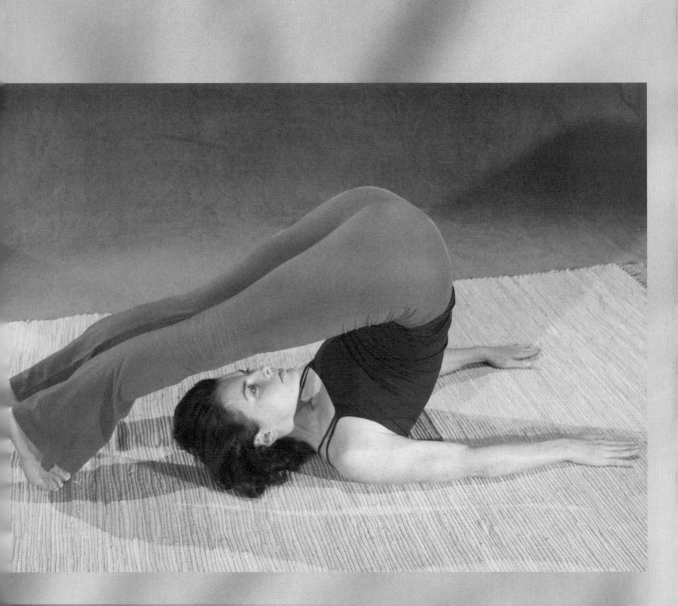

Meditation: Bring your attention to your genitals (root chakra)—which is easy to do, since you're actually looking at the root chakra area in this position! Softly breathe *prana* into this area and imagine energy flowing smoothly throughout this sexual region.

Double Wind Releasing Pose

Pavanamuktasana

Setup: Lie on your back with both knees bent. Hug your knees to your chest. Keep your head and shoulders on the floor as you pull your knees inward.

Duration: Hold for five full breaths.

Benefits: Stimulates the root chakra. Also releases tension in the lower back.

Modification: You can do one leg at a time if necessary.

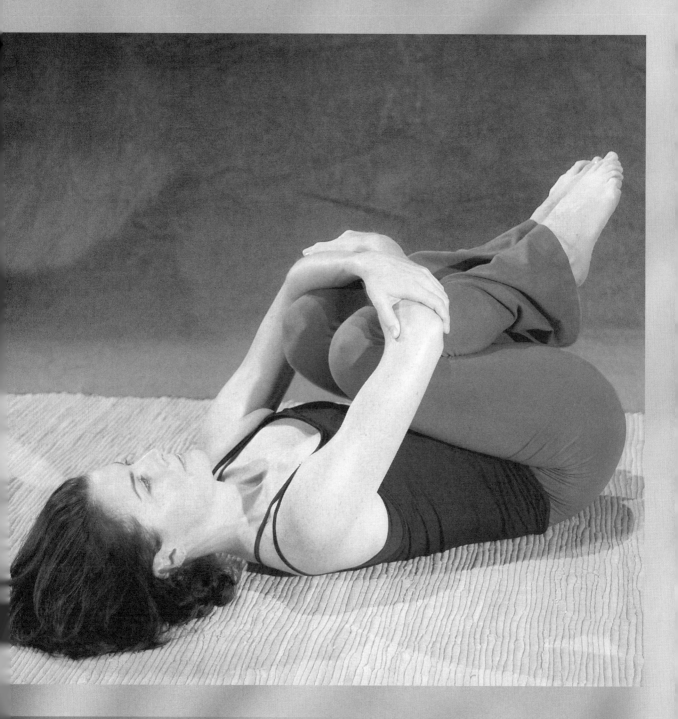

Meditation: Bring all of your attention to your pelvic floor, especially your root chakra. Softly breathe *prana* into that area and imagine energy flowing smoothly throughout this sexual region.

Lying Down Leg Raises

Supta Padangusthasana

Setup: Lie on your back and raise your right leg up. Grasp your calf with both hands. Exhale and lower your leg smoothly toward your right shoulder.

Duration: Hold this pose for five full breaths, exhale and gently release.

Benefits: This is an intense hip opener. You'll find several of the Divine Duets have this as one part of the partner pose, making it a way to prepare for the more advanced sexual positions.

Modification: If reaching your leg is difficult, use a strap.

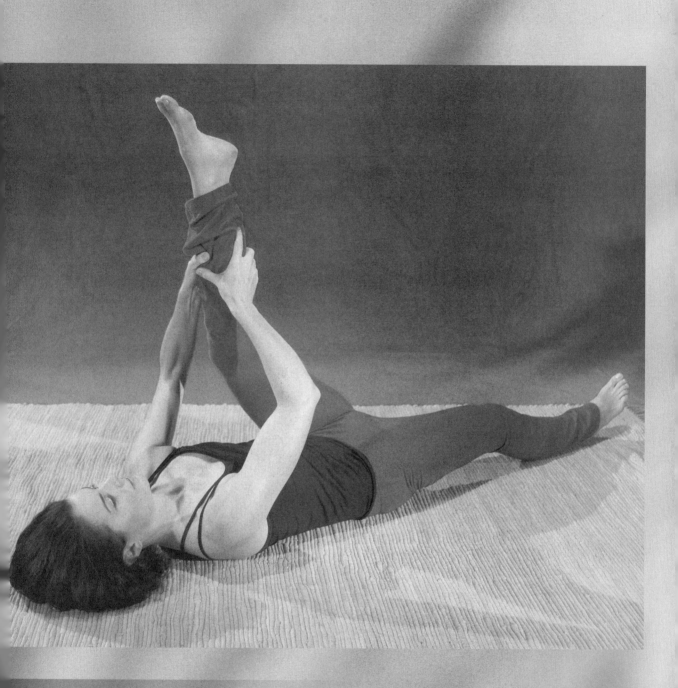

Meditation: Focus your thoughts on your hamstrings and breathe deeply and slowly. Obtaining flexibility here will be useful in the poses to come.

Fish Pose

Matsyasana

Setup: Lie on your back with your legs relaxed and straight on the floor. Inhale, lift your pelvis slightly off the floor, and slide your hands, palms down, below your butt. Then rest your butt on the backs of your hands—don't lift it off your hands as you perform this pose. Be sure to tuck your forearms and elbows close to the sides of your torso. Inhale and press your forearms and elbows firmly against the floor. With an inhale, lift your upper torso and head away from the floor. Then release your head back onto the floor. The crown of your head ideally rests on the floor. There should be a minimal amount of weight on your head to avoid crunching your neck.

Duration: Hold for five full breaths. Release with an exhalation and lower your torso and head to the floor.

Benefits: Fish Pose is a non-strenuous heart chakra opener, which means if you are seemingly too tired for sex, performing this pose takes minimal energy and helps restore your sexual vigor.

Modification: The back-bending position in *Matsyasana* can be difficult for beginning students. Perform the pose with your back supported on a thickly rolled blanket. Be sure to rest your head comfortably on the floor.

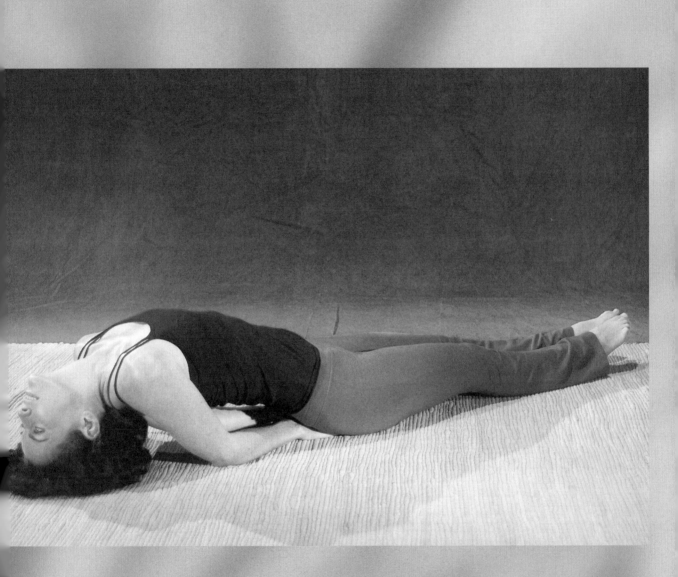

Meditation: Fish pose is a subtle inversion, which means lots of *prana* flows towards your crown chakra. Envision yourself with clear thoughts, articulate speech and a peaceful demeanor.

Supine Angle Pose

Supta Baddha Konasana

Setup: Lie flat on your back and bring the soles of your feet together while letting your knees fall open. Rest your hands on your lower belly.

Duration: Rest in this pose for three full minutes, breathing calmly.

Benefits: In women, this pose helps ease the pain of menstrual cramps. It also relaxes the vagina wall muscles, enhancing sexual pleasure. In men, this pose helps restore energy in the genitals, making it ideal to do before sex.

Modification: If your knees are tight, don't feel you have to make them touch the ground.

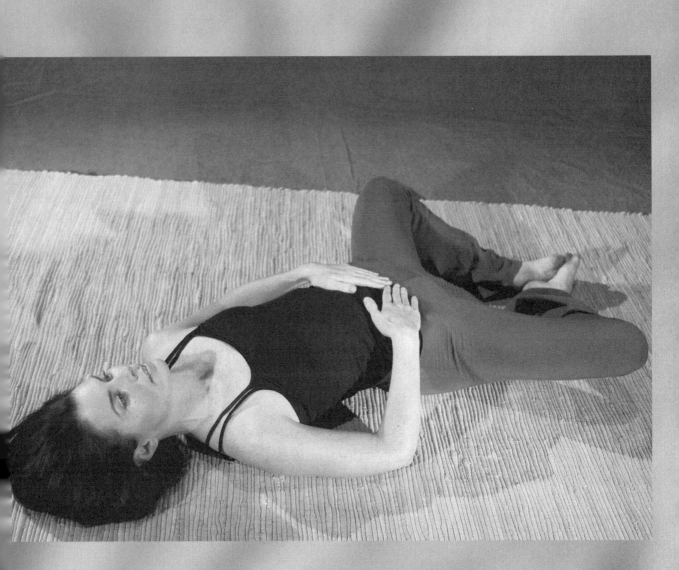

Meditation: Your hands are touching your sacral chakra, which is the area of the body that houses most of the female sexual organs. Focus all your attention on the sacral chakra, opening and stimulating the area. Imagine *prana* swirling effortlessly around the lower abdomen, stimulating and relaxing the entire zone.

Divine Duets

Divine Duets
Divine Duets
Divine Duets
Divine Duets

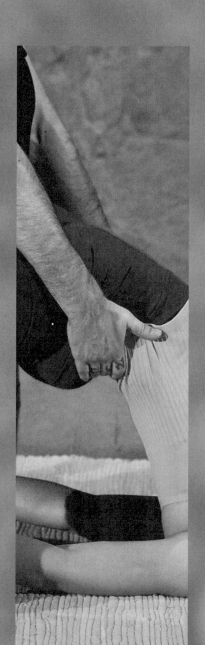

Have you heard the saying, "Partners who sweat together stay together"? Well, here is a chance to prove it right. The following are fifteen partner yoga postures that are directly adapted from the Kama Sutra. In the Duets, lovers perform an erotic yoga dance that's not only fun and sexy, it's healthy too. These postures invigorate the body, balance out hormonal levels and improve moods. The Duets are in no particular order, so you can jump around and pick postures you feel are appropriate to your fitness level. Some of the poses are for very experienced yogis only, so just take them in for now and use them as inspiration. I highly recommend performing the Glowing Solo poses first, as a warmup. Take the poses as far as you and your partner are ready to go. Be sure to maintain your *Ujjayi* breathing while attempting these poses and don't feel pressure to master them all at once.

The Clasping Position

Her Setup: Lie on your back. When your partner is in position, wrap your legs around his torso. Bring the soles of your feet together or cross your ankles behind his back.

Benefits: This pose is a gentle hip opener as well as a good stimulant for the root chakra.

His Setup: Lie on your belly between your partner's legs, with your legs straight and toes curled under, supporting your weight on your hands and toes. Press your hips down as you simultaneously extend your upper body up off the floor. (This is traditionally known as Cobra Pose.) Both of your legs are together and your arms are pressing your upper body into a mini backbend.

Benefits: This position stretches the upper chest, opening the heart chakra and strengthening the middle back muscles.

Duration: Hold this pose for up to 60 seconds.

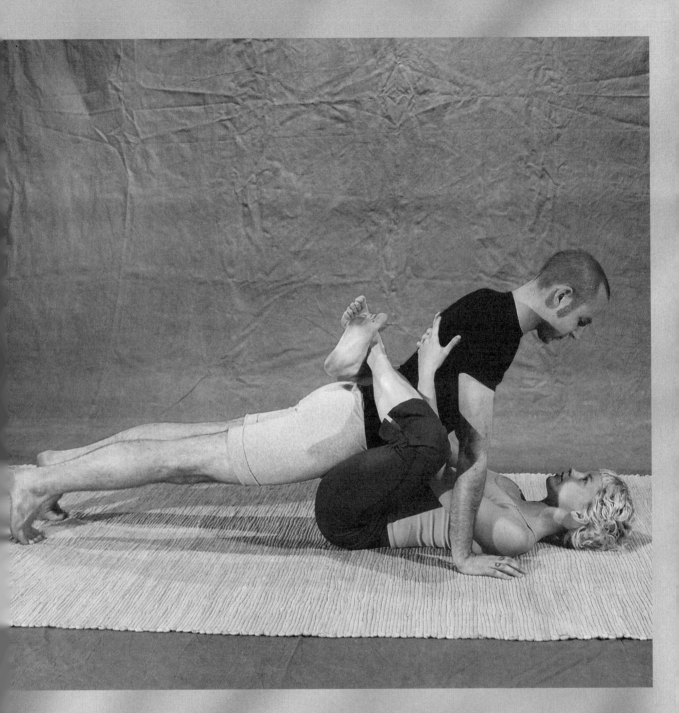

Partner Meditation: Bring your attention to both root

chakras—they are physically touching. Visualize the heat of this area, swirling up the spine, coating it with relaxation and health.

Wife of Indra

Her Setup: Lie on your back with your arms relaxed by your sides, legs straight up—your body forms a perfect 90-degree angle. Exhale, squeeze abdominal muscles and bring both legs up and overhead. At first, your toes should touch the floor behind your head, but as the pose intertwines, your legs will form a 45-degree angle. The knees can be straight or slightly bent. Be sure to keep the chin away from the chest, keep your abdominals pulled in and maintain an even flow of breath. Once your partner finds his position, rest your butt against his hips.

Benefits: This pose releases tension in the lower back. It also stretches the lower back muscles and hamstrings.

His Setup: Kneel on the floor with your knees six to eight inches apart and hands at your hips. Inhale and stretch the spine up, so your ribcage feels lifted off your waist. Exhale, and slowly release your head back, as if you're getting a shampoo. Continue bending your spine and pressing your hips forward. Place your right hand on your right heel, your left hand on your left heel. Try to keep your mouth closed and your eyes open and be sure to maintain a calm breath.

Benefits: This pose opens the heart chakra for improved breathing. It also strengthens the back muscles.

Duration: Try to hold this pose for 60 seconds.

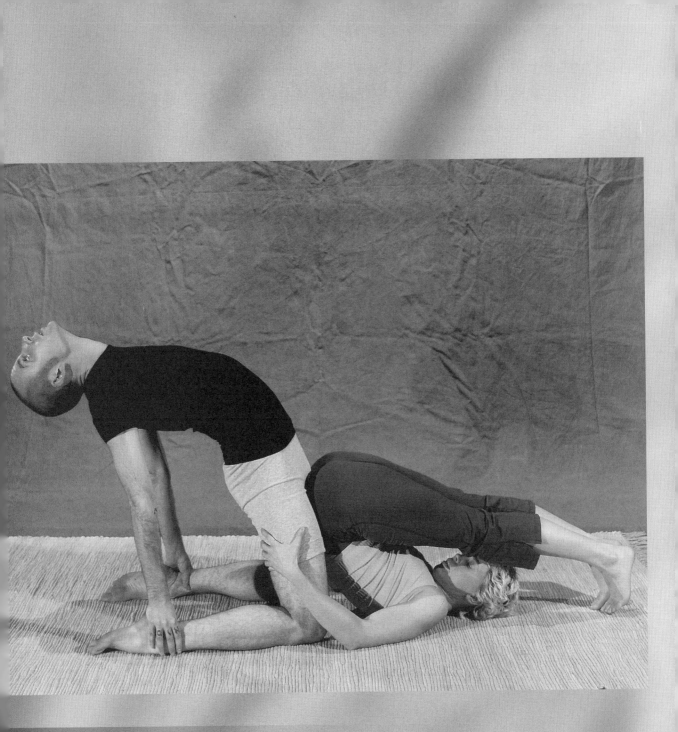

Partner Meditation: Feel each other's heartbeat as the woman brings her attention to her root chakra and the man brings his attention to his heart chakra.

The White Tiger Tao

Her Setup: Lie on your belly with your legs apart and feet flexed. Your inner knees are pressed against the floor and you're resting your upper body on your forearms. Feeling an intense stretch in the inner thigh means you're doing the pose right. Breathe calmly and evenly.

Benefits: This pose is an incredible relief for tight hips and knees.

His Setup: Press your belly against your partner's lower back and straddle her from behind. Your inner knees either press against her outer knees or simply toward the floor, depending on your leg length. Be sure to flex your feet (this protects the thigh muscles from strain). Dare to rock your body slowly up and down to find the perfect fit.

Benefits: This pose is an incredible relief for tight hips and knees.

Duration: Try to hold this pose for at least 60 seconds. If you are comfortable, you can hold it for up to five minutes.

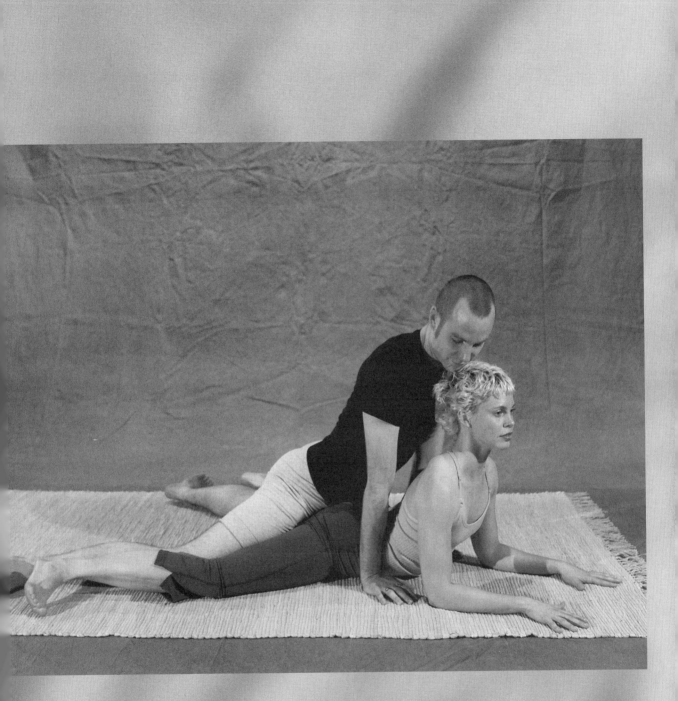

Partner Meditation: Try to synchronize your breathing
and bring all attention the sacral chakra. Imagine that area buzzing
with energy.

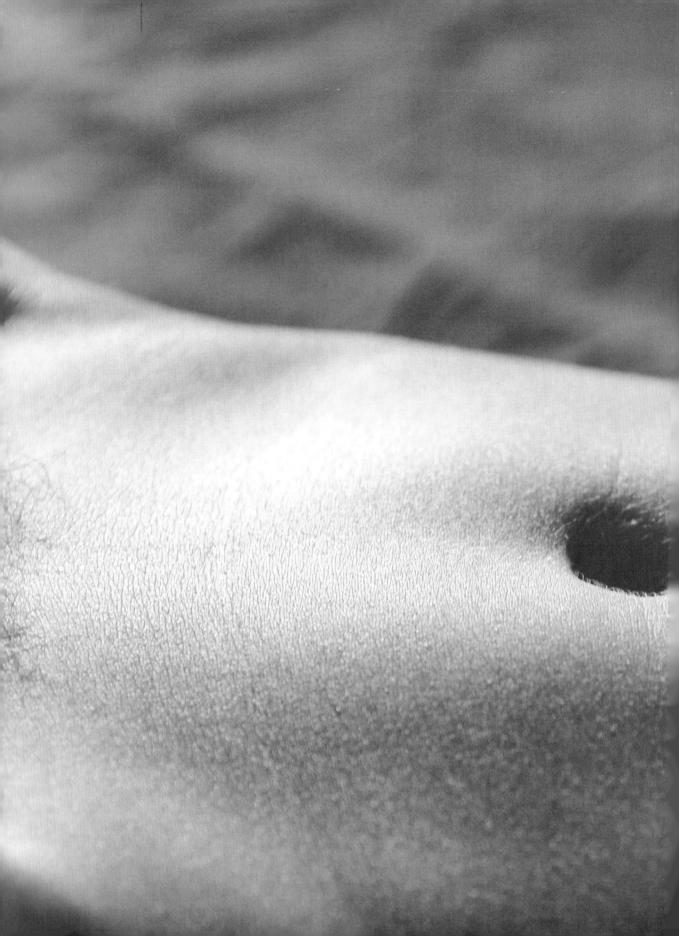

The Sacral Chakra

Consciousness of sexuality and sexual choices is related to the sacral chakra. Located approximately two fingers below the navel, this chakra is home to most of the sexual organs for women.

If this chakra is understimulated: Men and women may be obsessed with thoughts of sex or be emotionally explosive. Blockage in this area for women may lead to gynecological problems.

If this chakra is open: Since most of the female sexual organs reside here, sacral openness for women promotes the ability to freely flow with emotion and to feel and reach out to others sexually. For men, openness here translates to confidence in their ability to relate to others.

Kama's Wheel

His Setup: Sit on the floor with the soles of your feet together and your back tall and straight.

Benefits: This pose is a gentle hip opener and the added weight of your partner's body allows you to go more deeply into the stretch.

Her Setup: Gently sit on top of your partner with the soles of your feet together. Lean your back against his chest and help his knees push toward the floor by pressing open your own knees. Interlock your fingers around his feet if possible and have him interlock his fingers around your feet.

Benefits: This pose stretches the muscles surrounding the knees as well as the inner thigh muscles.

Duration: Hold this pose for up to two minutes.

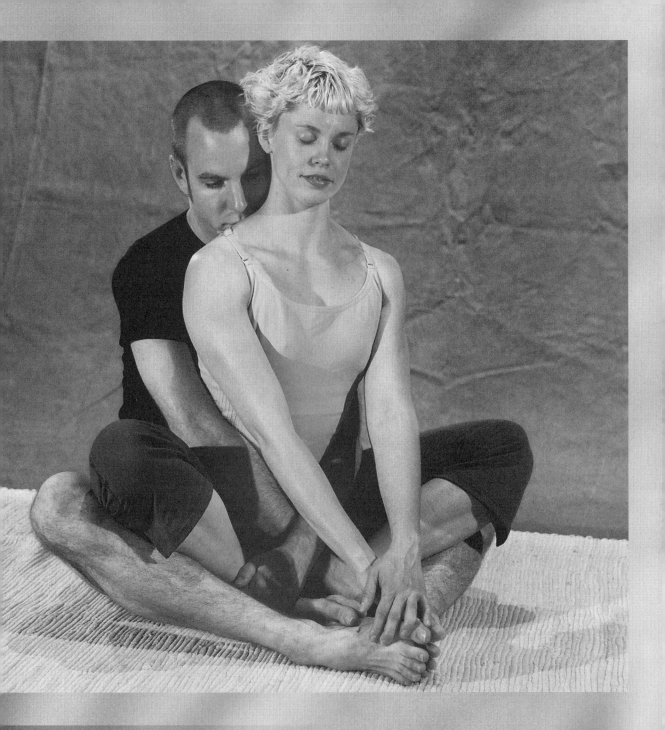

Partner Meditation: Feel for each other's heartbeat and then imagine your hearts circulating life force into the three sexual chakras— the root, sacral and heart.

Face-to-Face Pose

Her Setup: Lie on your back with legs three feet apart and relax. Reach your arms overhead.

Benefits: This pose is passive and meditative. It lets your body surrender completely to the earth for deep relaxation.

His Setup: Lie on top of your partner. Press your hips gently down toward her hips and lift your upper body into a mini backbend. Your legs are together and straight, and you're up on your toes. Reach up and clasp her hands securely. This takes a lot of back strength and balance.

Benefits: This position stretches the upper chest, opening the heart chakra and strengthening the mid-back muscles.

Duration: Hold for up to two minutes.

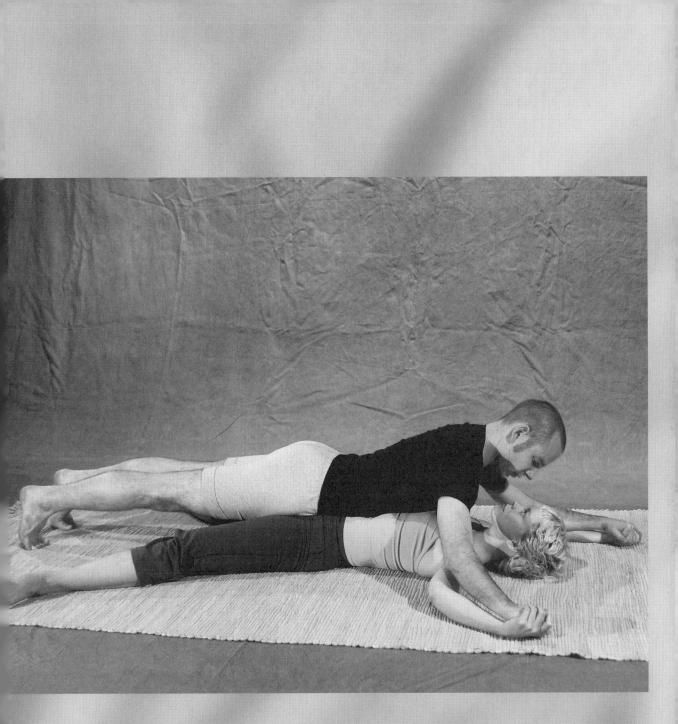

Partner Meditation: Since the sacral and root chakras are
pressed up against each other, bring all attention to those two areas. As
you inhale, attempt to direct the breath toward the sacral and root
chakras and imagine a cleansing force washing away unwanted stress.

Anango-Rango Position

Her Setup: Lie on your back and bend your knees, placing your heels close to your butt, hip distance apart. Place your hands under your shoulders, fingers pointing toward your feet. On an exhale, use your leg strength to lift your hips off the floor and use your arm strength to press your head and shoulders up. It feels like an inverted push-up. Try to keep your butt muscles relaxed by using only your leg and arm strength.

Benefits: This pose—one of the most challenging backbends—is filled with benefits. For one, you open and stimulate the heart and sacral chakras, which is great for breathing and for your emotional health. Second, this pose strengthens all muscles of the back, from the coccyx to the neck. Third, it improves arm and leg strength.

His Setup: Stand in front of your partner, looking down at her belly and hips. Reach around her lower back and interlace all ten fingers behind her lower back. Gently arch your back into a standing backbend, using her hips as resistance. You can bend your knees or lift her feet to find the perfect fit.

Benefits: This position stretches the upper chest, opening the heart chakra and strengthening the mid-back muscles. It also stretches the hip flexors.

Duration: Hold for 30 to 60 seconds.

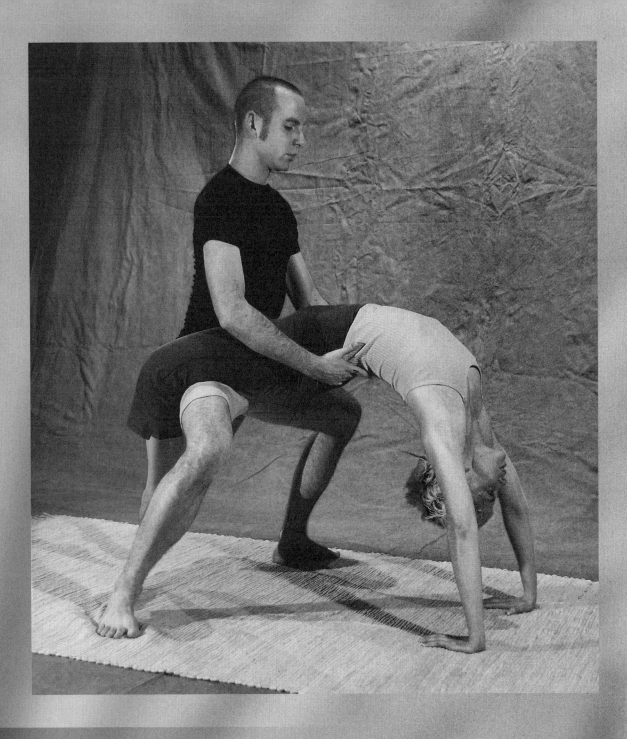

Partner Meditation: Both partners need to simply focus on breathing deeply. This will help you stay calm and in the present moment.

The Congress of the Cow

Her Setup: Position yourself on your hands and knees. Your knees should be directly under your hips and your hands should be shoulder distance apart. Look up and arch your back downward. This is called Cow Pose.

Benefits: This pose relaxes the lower back muscles and helps strengthen the abdominals.

His Setup: Kneel behind your partner with knees between her legs. Grab onto her hips as you press your hips towards her and gently bend back into a moderate Camel Pose.

Benefits: This pose releases tension in the chest, strengthens the mid-back muscles and stretches the hip flexors.

Duration: Hold for up to 60 seconds.

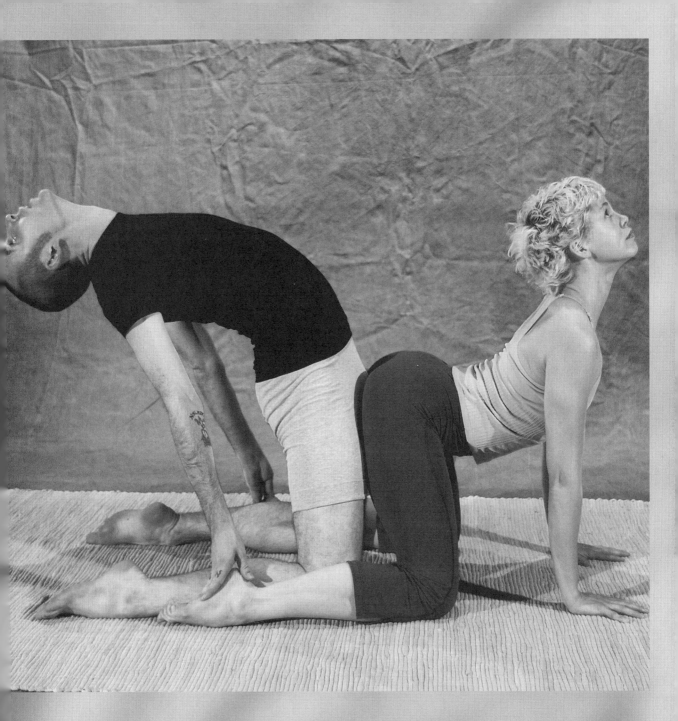

Partner Meditation:

The woman should meditate on her stable, grounded stance. Imagine feeling this sturdy in your emotional life as well. The man should visualize his heart expanding, allowing for more compassion, love and emotional health to enter into his life.

Driving the Peg Home

Her Setup: Stand with feet together, inner edges touching, and reach around, grabbing your partner's hips from behind with both hands. Strongly press your hips into his—this will keep you stable and balanced. Lift your torso up and off your waist, and lean back. The energy moves up and back while your feet are well-grounded to the floor.

Benefits: This pose opens the heart and sacral chakras simultaneously, for improved circulation within the female sexual organs and an increase in emotional well-being.

His Setup: Stand with feet together, inner edges touching, and reach around, grabbing your partner's hips from behind with both hands. Strongly press your hips into hers—this will keep you stable and balanced. Lift your torso up and off your waist and lean back. The energy moves up and back while your feet stay grounded on the floor.

Benefits: This pose opens the heart and sacral chakras simultaneously, for improved circulation and breathing capacity and an increase in emotional well-being.

Duration: Hold for up to two minutes.

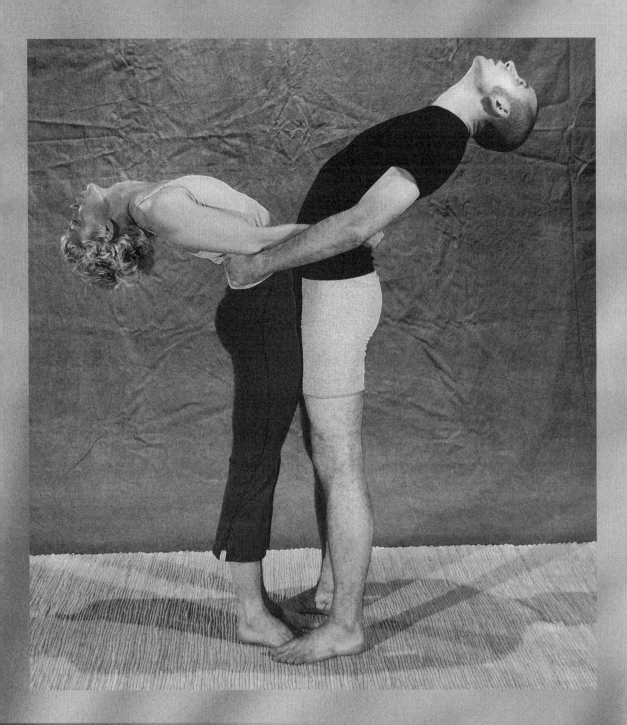

Partner Meditation: Notice how both partners have their feet firmly fixed to the ground while their heads are reaching toward the heavens, and each partner is supporting the other. This is a great metaphor for being rooted in reality but focused on your dreams, with a big bonus—the added support of each other.

The Mill Vanes

Her Setup: Lie flat on your back and bring the soles of your feet together, letting your knees fall open. Rest your hands on your partner's butt.

Benefits: This pose helps ease the pain of menstrual cramps because it relaxes the abdominal region. It also gently opens the hips.

His Setup: Start in the Spread Leg Forward Bend Pose (see page 32) and walk your hands away from your body until your belly touches the floor between your partner's legs, then prop your upper body up with your arms. Maintain the wide stance the entire pose. The insides of both feet and knees are pressing against the ground. Gently attempt to bring your hips as close to the floor as possible. It is important to enter into this pose very slowly, so take your time and breathe into every inch of the movement.

Benefits: You really challenge your hip and groin muscles, which makes this pose great for improving flexibility in the inner thighs.

Duration: This pose can be held for up to five minutes.

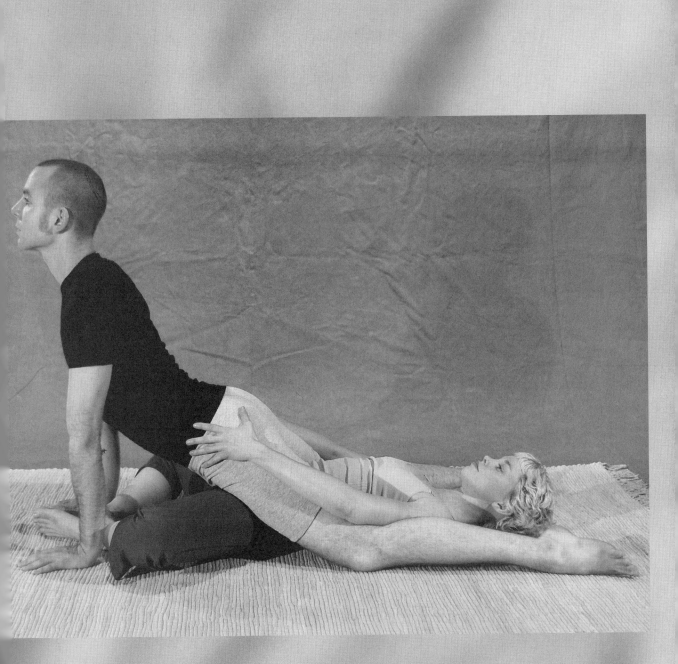

Partner Meditation: Since you are not facing each other, try to synchronize your breath. Once it's synchronized, try to extend it, by inhaling and exhaling slower, deeper and longer.

The Ascending Position

His Setup: Lie on your back with your legs relaxed, straight on the floor. Inhale, lift your pelvis slightly off the floor, and slide your hands, palms down, below your butt. Then rest your butt on the backs of your hands—don't lift the hips off your hands as you perform this pose. Be sure to tuck your forearms and elbows in close to the sides of your torso. Inhale and press your forearms and elbows firmly against the floor. With an inhale, lift your upper torso and head away from the floor. Then release your head back onto the floor. The crown of your head ideally rests on the floor. There should be a minimal amount of weight on your head to avoid crunching your neck.

Benefits: This is a non-strenuous heart chakra opener, so it requires minimal energy. It helps make for deeper, more efficient breathing.

Her Setup: Straddle the hips of your partner, with your heels adjacent to his upper thighs. You are in a supported Hero's Pose. At first, sit upright with a straight spine and settle into the posture. When ready, inhale and extend your torso forward, draping your body over your knees, towards your partner's heart. Keep your hips down and feel the extension of the spine and the stretch in both knees.

Benefits: Forward Hero's Pose is especially great for improving knee flexibility, which is vital in many of the Sacred Sex positions.

Duration: Hold anywhere between 60 seconds and up to five minutes.

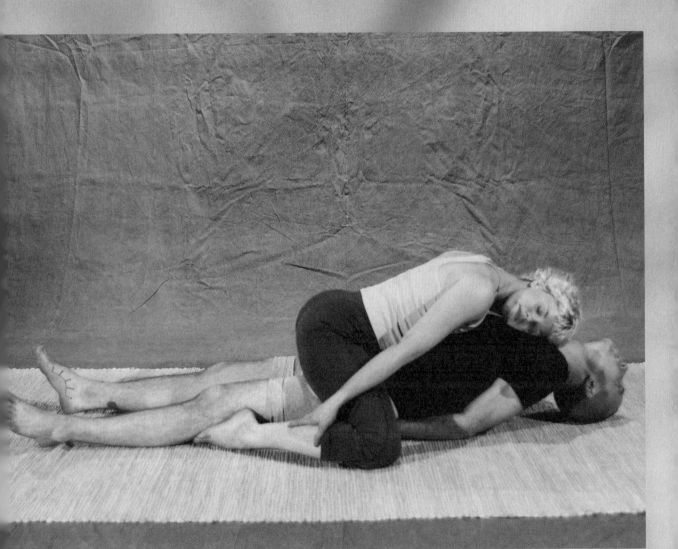

Partner Meditation: Concentrate on the "heat" of human touch. Observe how energy is transferred and feel the warm flow between the two beings.

The Arc

Her Setup: Lie on your back with your arms relaxed by your sides, knees bent and feet planted hip width apart or wider—whatever distance feels most comfortable. On your next exhale, push your hips up off the ground toward your partner. As the position evolves, you may want to place your hands on your lower back, hoisting your hips up even higher. Breathe deeply and feel your spine lengthen in opposition.

Benefits: This pose gently heats the body. It opens the heart center for improved intimacy with one's self and others. It also aids in the release of bottled-up emotion.

His Setup: Kneel with your butt on your heels, facing your partner, like in Prayer Squat. She is on her back and your knees are between her legs. Now, slide your hips up to meet your partner's. Splay your feet out to the sides slightly, giving you a better grip on the floor. If you like, lean your body forward, trying to drape your body over hers.

Benefits: This opens the root chakra, and rests the sacral chakra while the heart chakra is in neutral. All energy goes directly toward the root, releasing unwanted stress in the sexual organs.

Duration: Hold for up to two minutes.

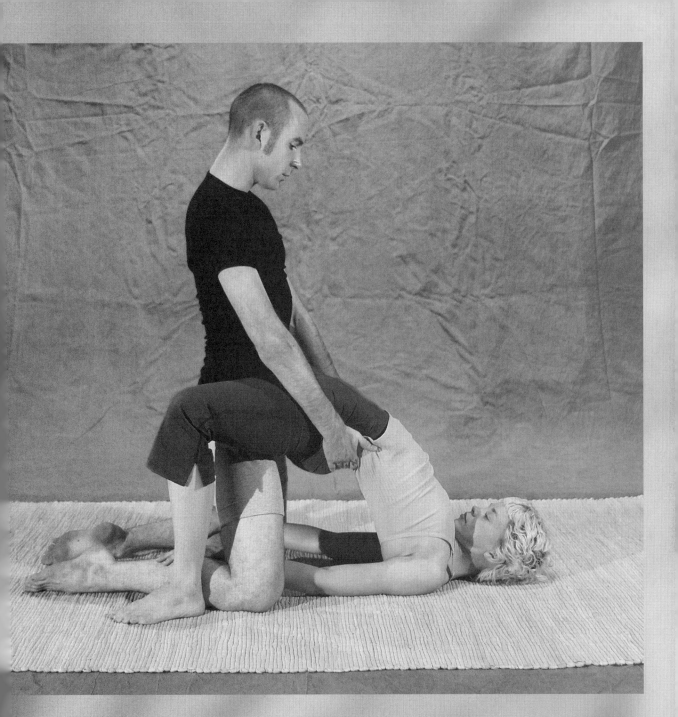

Partner Meditation: Balancing in this pose will be a challenge for both partners, so bring your focus to the idea of balance by trying to remain as still as possible.

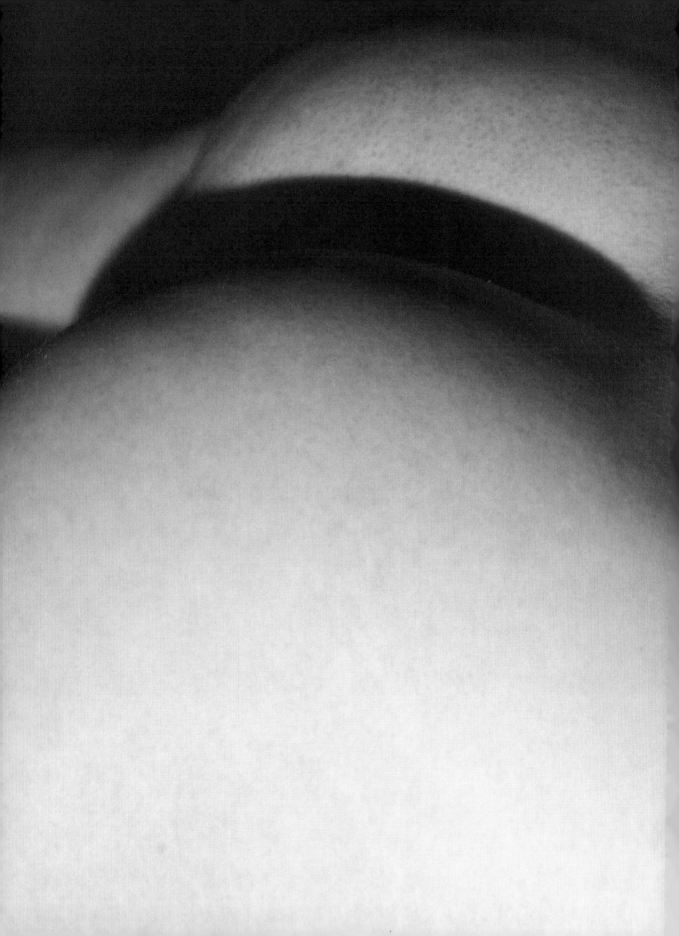

The Root Chakra

The root chakra is also called the first chakra, because it governs the primal concept of self-preservation. The perineum—the area midway between the genitals and the anus—is its exact, very intimate, location. In Eastern teachings it is given the name *Muladahra*, meaning root or support, because the other six central chakras all stem from this one.

If this chakra is understimulated: Both men and women tend to feel sexually inferior, undesirable or frustrated. Men may experience impotence.

If this chakra is open: Great sexual stamina, energy and a lack of inhibition. A natural Viagra effect!

The Twining Position

Her Setup: Lie on your back and raise your left leg. Hold the big toe of your left foot with the first two fingers of your left hand. Exhale and pull your leg smoothly toward your left shoulder. The pressure of your partner's torso will aid in deepening the stretch.

Benefits: This pose is a great hamstrings stretch and hip opener. It also massages the abdomen for better digestion.

His Setup: Face your partner and bring your left leg up toward her shoulder. Hold the big toe of your left foot with the first two fingers of your left hand. Your right leg can be bent if necessary.

Benefits: This pose is a great hamstrings stretch and hip opener. It also massages the abdomen for better digestion.

Duration: Hold for up to two minutes.

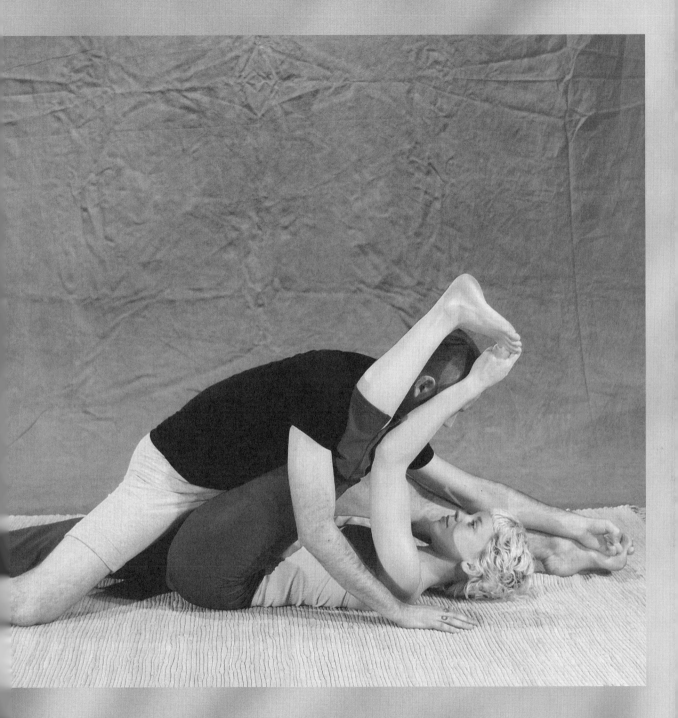

Partner Meditation: Both partners are essentially feeling the same hamstrings challenge. For this meditation, imagine breathing relief into each other's hamstrings.

The Amazon

His Setup: Lie on your back with both knees bent in toward your shoulders. Keep your head and shoulders on the floor. Your aim is to bring your knees to your shoulders and be passive.

Benefits: This pose brings energy to the root chakra, which releases unwanted tension in the hips and the root chakra.

Her Setup: Stand with feet six inches apart, bend your knees and squat down over your partner. With your legs outside his knees, rest your butt down on his hips. His knees are in a fairly narrow stance. Comfortably clasp hands with your partner for better balance and try to synchronize your breathing.

Benefits: This pose directs a great deal of energy toward the root chakra, which will relax the pelvic floor muscles. It also simultaneously strengthens and stretches the knee joints.

Duration: Hold for up to three minutes.

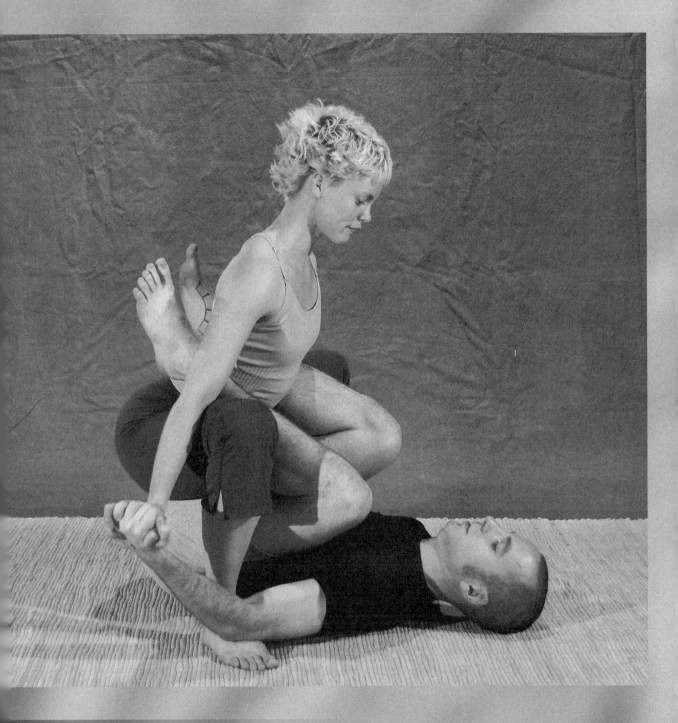

Partner Meditation: The root chakra is the focal point for both partners, so bring your attention and breath there and feel the life force cleansing, strengthening and relaxing the entire area.

The Trapeze

His Setup: Sit in a partial squat with knees apart, propped up on the edge of a bed or couch. You'll want to be holding on to your partner's hips as the pose progresses.

Benefits: This pose directs a great deal of energy toward the root chakra, which will relax the pelvic floor muscles. It also simultaneously strengthens and stretches the knee joints.

Her Setup: Sit on top of your partner, straddling him as if in Seated Angle Pose. If possible bring the soles of your feet together. Now slowly drop your head back and arch your spine down toward the floor. You should feel as though you are inverted and you're relying on your partner for stability.

Benefits: This pose is a subtle inversion, which improves circulation in the entire body.

Duration: Hold for up to two minutes.

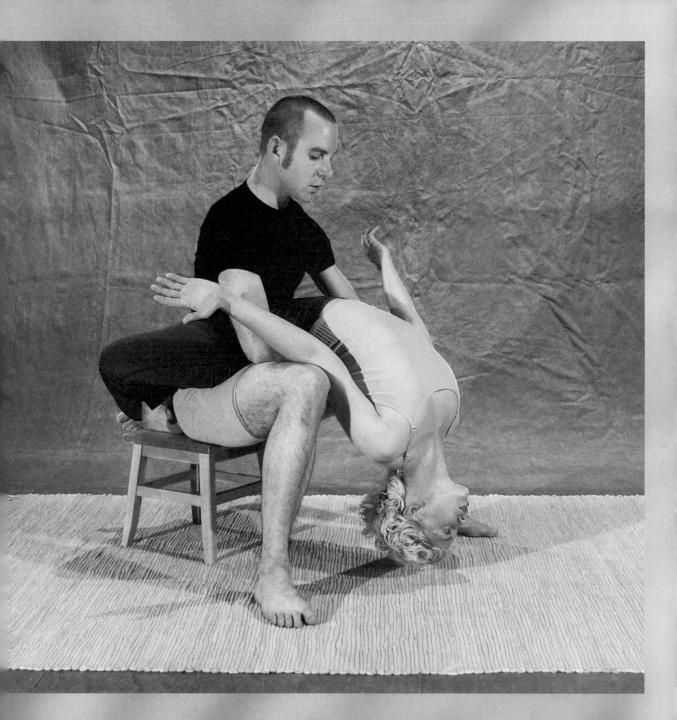

Partner Meditation: The root chakra is the focal point for
both partners, so bring your attention and breath there and feel the life
force cleansing, strengthening and relaxing the entire area.

The Surprise

His Setup: Stand behind your partner, with your legs approximately one foot apart. Knees can be bent or straight. Press your body against your partner's butt and hug your arms around her waist. Look to the sky and arch back.

Benefits: This pose challenges balance and stretches the hip flexors.

Her Setup: Stand with your back to your partner and bend over at the waist. Relax your upper body in this forward bend position and simply breathe.

Benefits: This pose releases tension in the lower back and stretches the hamstrings.

Duration: Hold for up to five minutes.

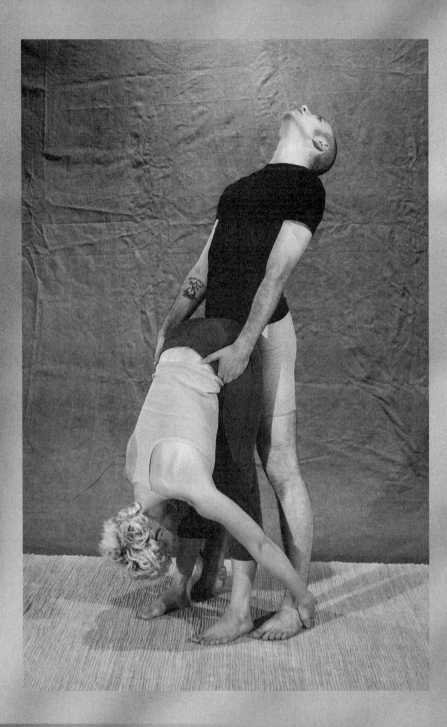

Partner Meditation: In the Surprise position, the man is very active while the woman is very passive. Meditate on these two opposi- tions. We tend to think that "active" is more strenuous and therefore "better," but actually passivity can be just as beneficial and challenging, as in this pose.

Sacred Sex

The Kama Sutra presents sex as sacred—essential to life, a gift from God, worthy of serious study. Now that you have practiced the solo and duet yoga poses, you are ready for the real thing: sexual positions from the Kama Sutra. These sexual positions promote fabulous sex, increase intimacy and add some zest to your life in general. The original Kama Sutra was written "to prevent the separation of the married pair." This, of course, is my deepest desire for you and your lover and the ultimate purpose of this section.

The Clasping Position

Her Setup: Lie on your back. When your lover is in position, wrap your legs around his torso. Bring the soles of your feet together behind his back or cross your ankles.

His Setup: Lie on your belly between your lover's legs, with your legs straight. Press your hips down as you simultaneously extend your upper body up off the bed. (This is traditionally known as Cobra Pose.) Both of your legs are together and your arms are pressing your upper body into a mini backbend.

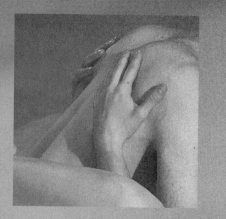 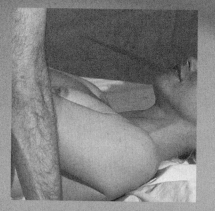 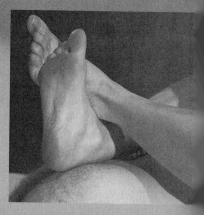

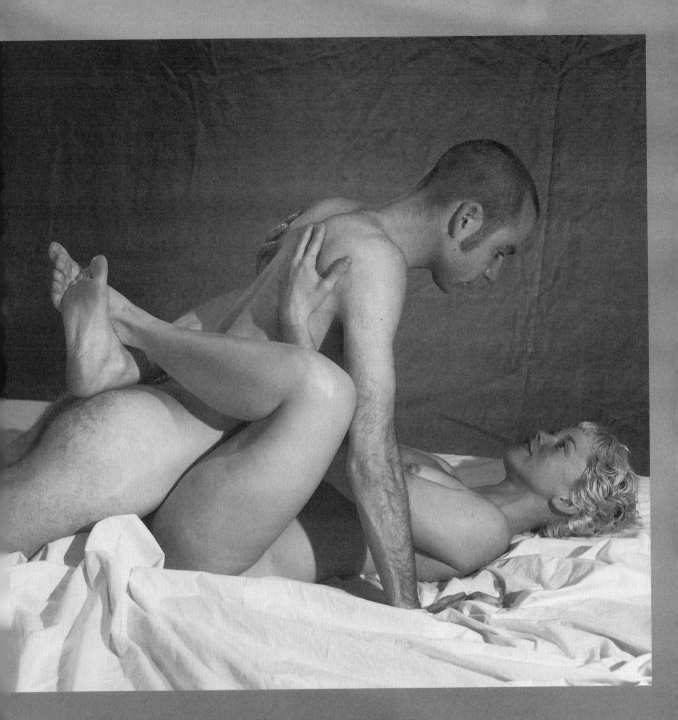

The pleasure of the pose: The Clasping Position is easy
to attain, making it perfect for all fitness levels. Man and woman are
face-to-face, which facilitates kissing, stroking and gazing into each
other's eyes.

Wife of Indra

Her Setup: Lie on your back with your arms relaxed by your sides, legs straight up—your body forms a perfect 90-degree angle. Exhale, squeeze your abdominal muscles and bring both legs up and overhead. At first, your toes should touch the bed behind your head, but as the pose intertwines, your legs will form a 45-degree angle. The knees can be straight or slightly bent. Be sure to keep the chin away from the chest, keep your abdominals pulled in and maintain an even flow of breath. Once your lover finds his position, rest your butt against his hips.

His Setup: Kneel in front of your lover with your knees six to eight inches apart and hands at your hips. Inhale and stretch the spine up, so your ribcage feels lifted off your waist. Exhale, and slowly release your head back, as if you're getting a shampoo. Continue bending your spine and pressing your hips forward, against your lover. Place your right hand on your right heel, your left hand on your left heel. Try to keep your mouth closed and your eyes open and be sure to maintain a calm breath.

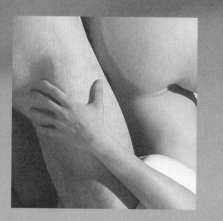 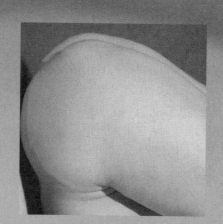 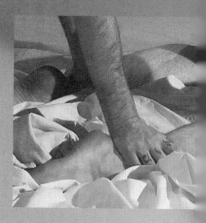

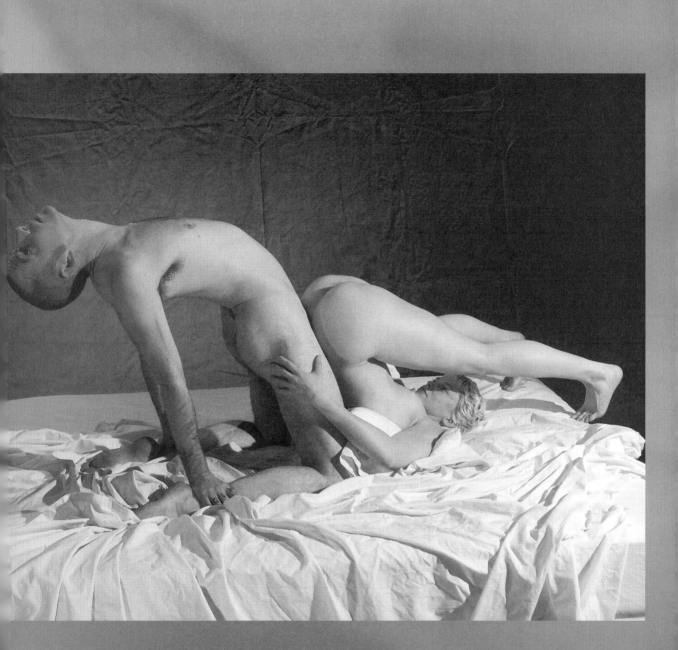

The pleasure of the pose: The woman's root chakra

tends to be very relaxed and open in this position, increasing her sexual pleasure.

The White Tiger Tao

Her Setup:
Lie on your belly with your legs apart and feet flexed. Your inner knees are pressed against the bed and you're resting your upper body on your forearms. Feeling an intense stretch in the inner thigh means you're doing the pose right. Breathe calmly and evenly.

His Setup:
Press your belly against your lover's lower back and straddle her from behind. Your inner knees either press against her outer knee or simply toward the bed, depending on your leg length. Be sure to flex your feet (this protects the thigh muscles from strain). Dare to rock your body slowly up and down to find the perfect fit.

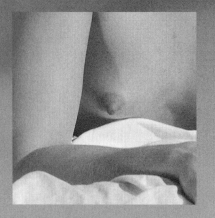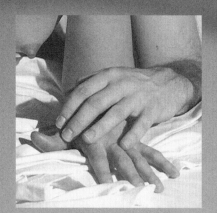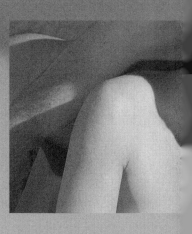

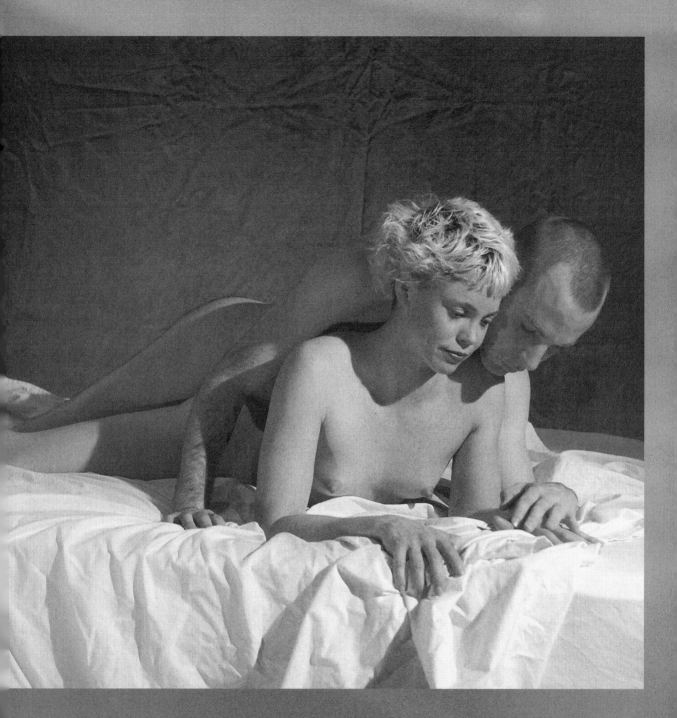

The pleasure of the pose: In this position, the man can illustrate his masculinity by penetrating deeply and aggressively, like a tiger in the wild.

Kama's Wheel

His Setup: Sit with the soles of your feet together and your back tall and straight.

Her Setup: Gently sit on top of your lover with the soles of your feet together. Lean your back against his chest and help his knees push down by pressing open your own knees. Interlock your fingers around his feet if possible and have him interlock his fingers around your feet.

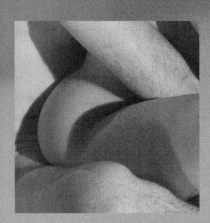
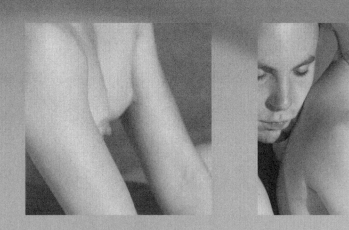

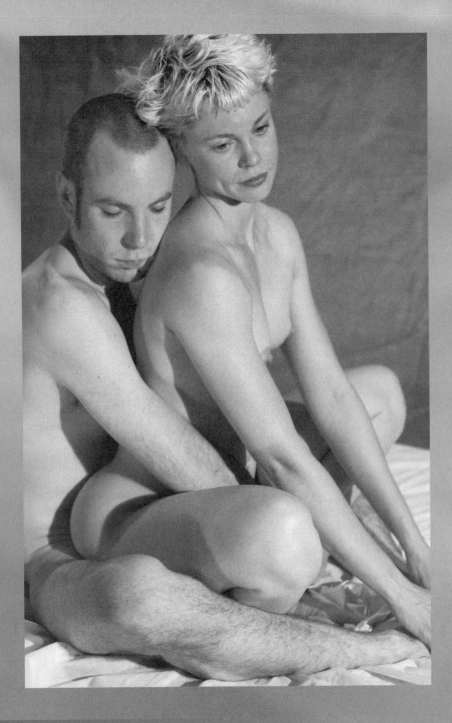

The pleasure of the pose: A legendary sexual position, it
is said that Kama's Wheel combines sex and meditation to bring us to a
higher level of awareness. This position is meant to help both lovers
obtain a balance of mind that is clear, calm and happy.

Face-to-Face Pose

Her Setup: Lie on your back with legs three feet apart and relax. Reach your arms overhead.

His Setup: Lie on top of your lover. Press your hips gently down toward her hips and lift your upper body into a mini backbend. Both of your legs are together and straight. Reach up and clasp her hands securely. This takes a lot of back strength and balance. Use your arms to control your thrusts as you pin her to the bed.

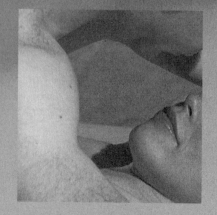
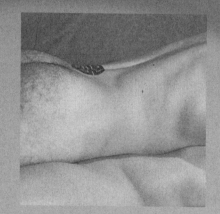
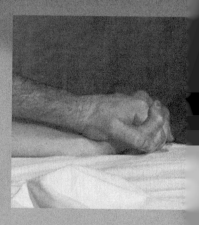

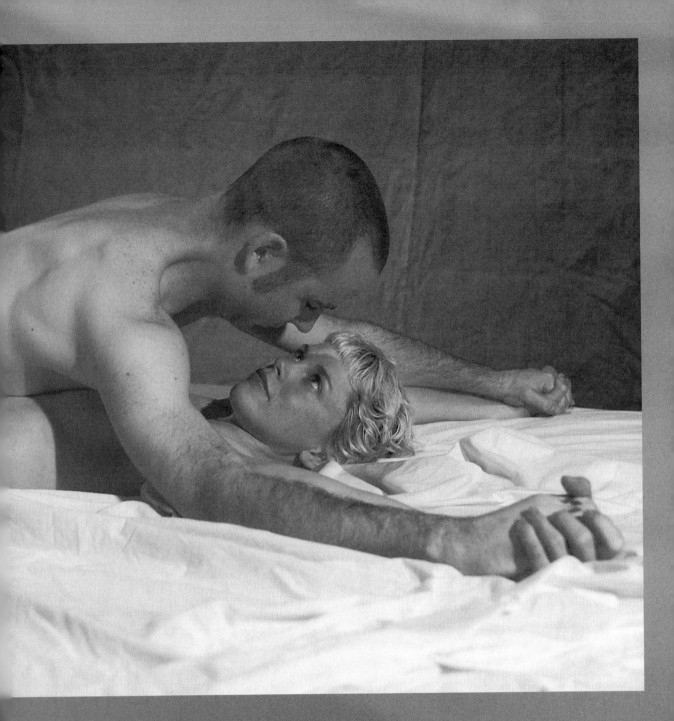

The pleasure of the pose: This is a classic and universal position. As stated in the Kama Sutra, "If the male be long-timed, the female loves him more. If he is short-timed, she is dissatisfied with him." This pose helps men avoid early ejaculation and thus be "long-timed."

Anango-Rango Position

Her Setup: Lie on your back and bend your knees, placing your heels close to your butt, hip distance apart. Place your hands under your shoulders, fingers pointing toward your feet. On an exhale, use your leg strength to lift your hips off the floor and use your arm strength to press your head and shoulders up. It feels like an inverted push-up. You can thrust your hips back and forth in this position, aiding in the sexual arousal.

His Setup: Situate yourself in front of your lover, so you are standing, looking down at her belly and hips. Reach around her and interlace all ten fingers behind her lower back, pressing up against her as you guide yourself in. You can lift her feet off the ground to find the perfect fit.

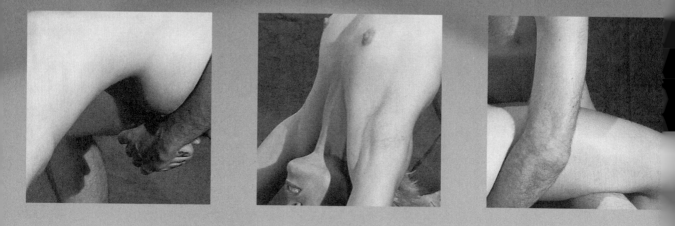

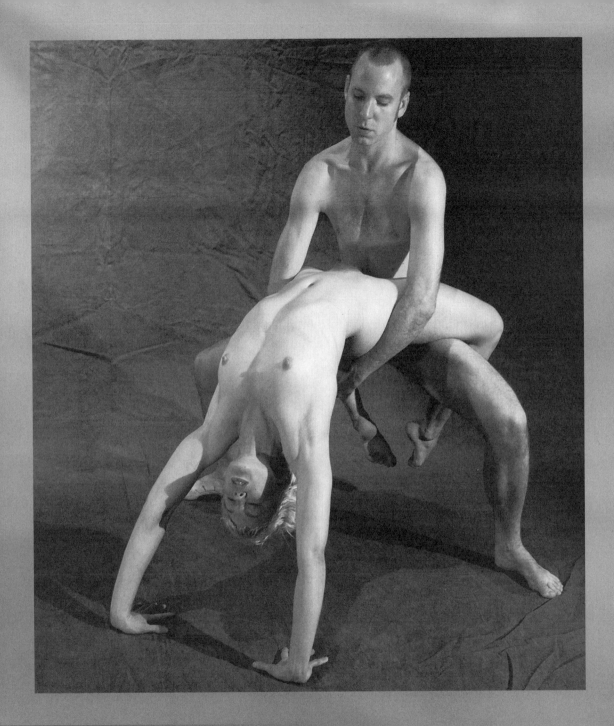

The pleasure of the pose: It's quite an accomplishment if you can pull this position off—acrobatics galore! According to the Kama Sutra, the excitement surrounding this pose is extraordinary and will give both the man and woman extreme pleasure and "bragging rights."

The Congress of the Cow

Her Setup: Position yourself on your hands and knees. Your knees should be directly under your hips and your hands should be shoulder distance apart.

His Setup: Kneel behind your lover with your knees between her legs. Exhale, and slowly release your head back, as if you're getting a shampoo. Continue bending your spine and pressing your hips forward, against your lover. Place your right hand on your right heel, your left hand on your left heel. Try to keep your mouth closed and your eyes open and be sure to maintain a calm breath.

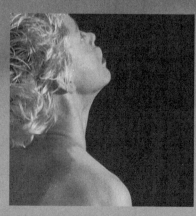
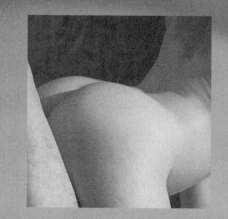
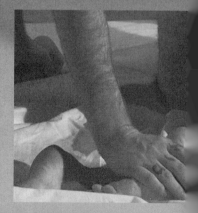

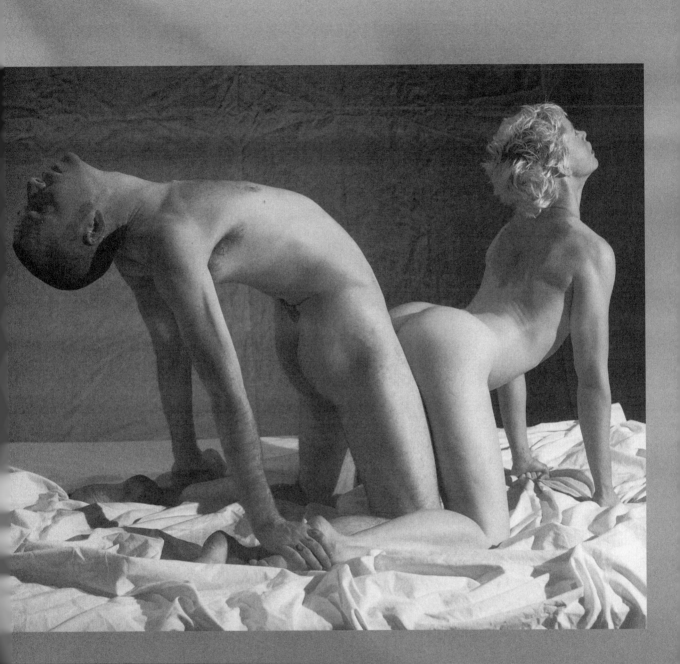

The pleasure of the pose: The man is able to penetrate
very deeply in this sexual position, making way for intense sensation for
both parties.

Driving the Peg Home

Her Setup: Stand with feet together, inner edges touching, and reach around, grabbing your lover's hips from behind with both hands. Strongly press your hips into his—this will keep you stable and balanced. Lift your torso up and off your waist, and lean back. The energy moves up and back while your feet are well-grounded to the floor.

His Setup: Stand with feet together, inner edges touching, and reach around, grabbing your lover's hips from behind with both hands. Strongly press your hips into hers—this will keep you stable and balanced. Lift your torso up and off your waist and lean back. The energy moves up and back while your feet stay grounded on the floor.

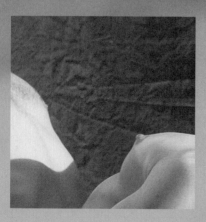
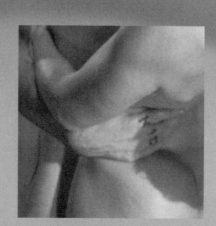
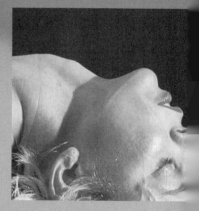

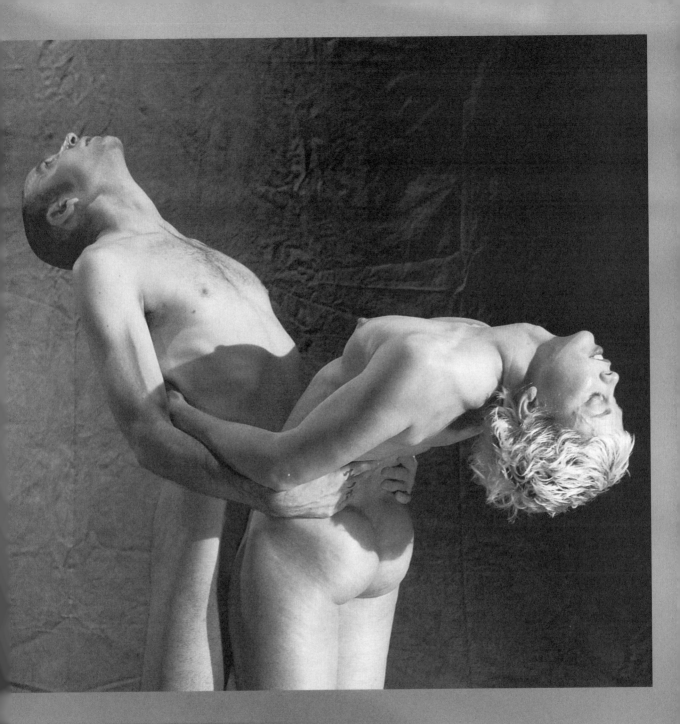

The pleasure of the pose: Not only is this posture one of the most beautiful, it's also considered the "unloading" pose. Because of the narrow stance and increased friction, men can reach full orgasm easily.

The Mill Vanes

Her Setup: Lie flat on your back and bring the soles of your feet together, letting your knees fall open. Rest your hands on your lover's butt.

His Setup: Start in the Spread Leg Forward Bend Pose and walk your hands away from your body until your belly touches the bed between your lover's legs, then prop your upper body up with your arms. Maintain the wide stance the entire pose. The insides of both feet and knees are pressing against the ground. Gently attempt to bring your hips as close to the bed as possible. It is important to enter into this pose very slowly, so take your time and breathe into every inch of the movement.

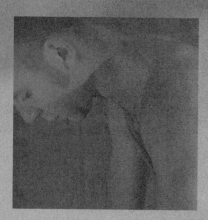
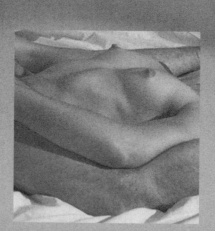
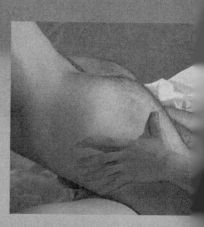

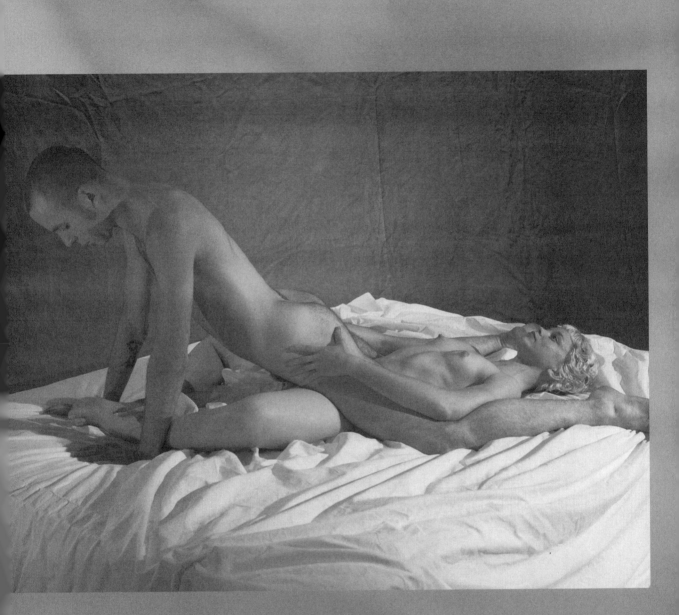

The pleasure of the pose: The angle of penetration is

very different than in other positions, which provides a greater variety of
sensation.

The Ascending Position

His Setup: Lie on your back with your legs relaxed and straight. Inhale, lift your pelvis slightly, and slide your hands, palms down, below your butt. Then rest your butt on the backs of your hands—don't lift the hips off your hands as you perform this pose. Be sure to tuck your forearms and elbows in close to the sides of your torso. Inhale and press your forearms and elbows firmly against the bed. With an inhale, lift your upper torso and head away from the bed. Then release your head back onto the bed. The crown of your head ideally rests on the bed. There should be a minimal amount of weight on your head to avoid crunching your neck.

Her Setup: Straddle the hips of your lover, with your heels adjacent to his upper thighs. You are in a supported Hero's Pose. At first, sit upright with a straight spine and settle into the posture. When ready, inhale and extend your torso forward, draping your body over your knees, towards your lover's heart. Keep your hips down and feel the extension of the spine and the stretch in both knees.

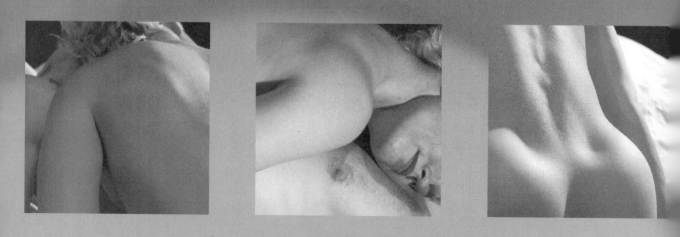

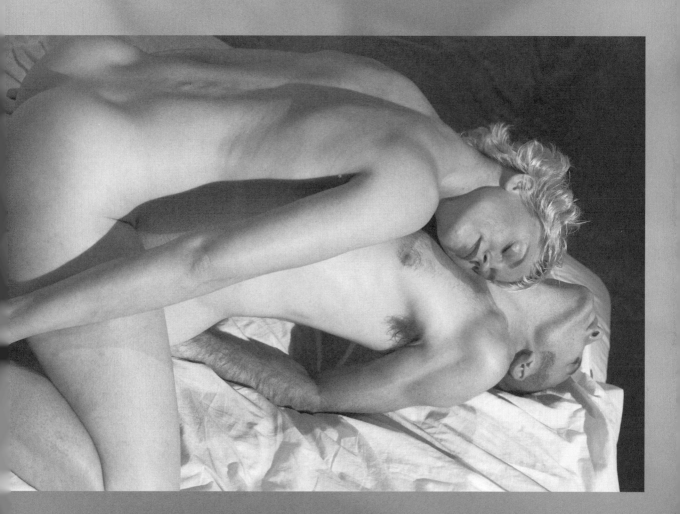

The pleasure of the pose: It's said to be great if the woman has been having a difficult time with orgasms. In this position, her posture is one that forces the vaginal walls to relax—plus, the woman, being on top, has control over the movements.

The Arc

Her Setup: Lie on your back with your arms relaxed by your sides, knees bent and feet planted hip width apart or wider—whatever distance suits the union best. On your next exhale, push your hips up off the bed toward your lover. As the position evolves, place your hands on your lower back or on the bed behind you, hoisting your hips up even higher. This will assist in the sexual merger. Breathe deeply and feel your spine lengthen in opposition.

His Setup: Kneel with your butt on your heels, facing your lover. She is on her back and your knees are between her legs. Now, slide your hips up to meet your lover's. Splay your feet out to the sides slightly, giving you a better grip on the bed. If you like, lean your body forward, as if trying to kiss your lover's breasts.

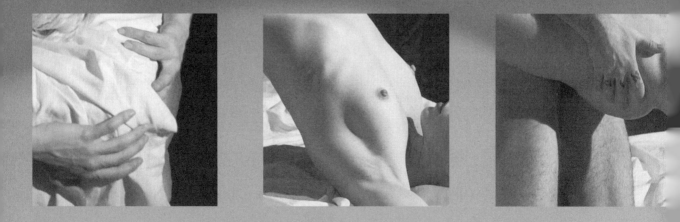

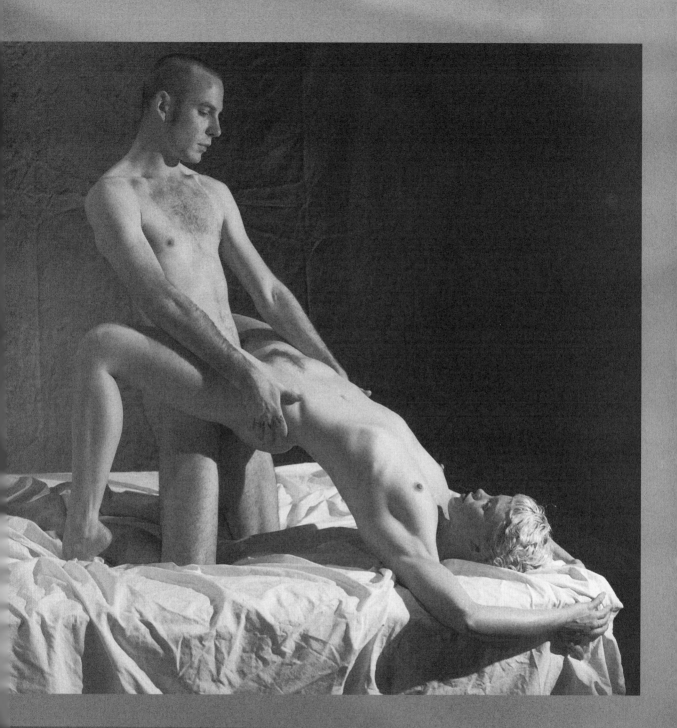

The pleasure of the pose: The pleasure received by

performing this position is legendary because the penis, with its deep penetration, is completely encompassed by the vaginal and abdominal zone of the woman. According to the Kama Sutra, men experience very powerful orgasms with this one.

The Twining Position

Her Setup: Lie on your back and raise your right leg. Hold the big toe of your right foot with the first two fingers of your right hand. Exhale and pull your leg smoothly toward your right shoulder. The pressure of your lover's torso will aid in deepening the stretch. You can let go of your foot once you find the pose.

His Setup: Face your lover and bring your right leg up toward her shoulder. Your left leg can be bent if necessary.

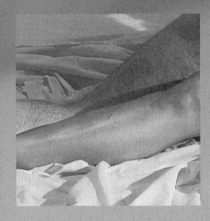 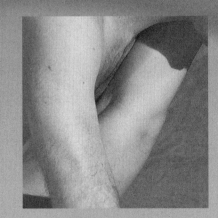 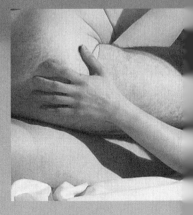

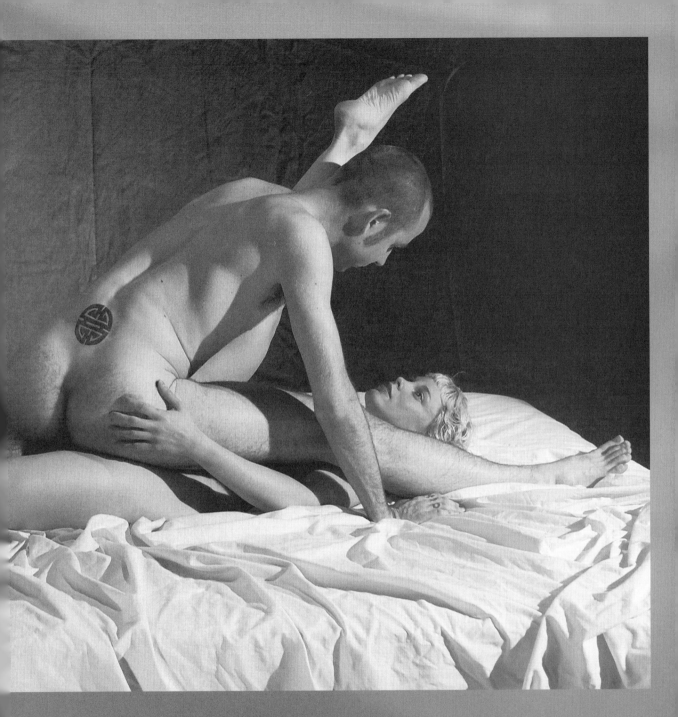

The pleasure of the pose: The physical challenge of
getting into this position makes the moment of entry more exciting.
Plus, entry tends to be easier, since the woman is very open.

The Amazon

His Setup: Lie on your back with both knees bent in toward your shoulders. Keep your head and shoulders on the bed. Your aim is to bring your knees to your shoulders and be passive.

Her Setup: Stand with feet six inches apart, bend your knees and squat down over your lover. With your legs outside his knees, rest your butt down on his hips. His knees are in a fairly narrow stance. Comfortably clasp hands with your lover by the sides of your connected bodies and breathe.

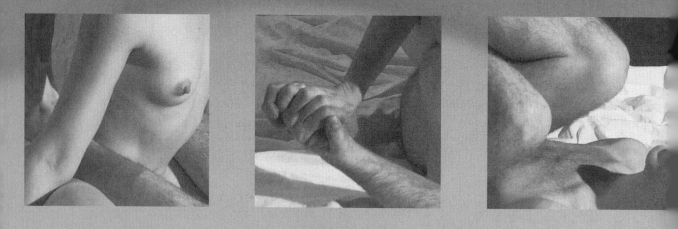

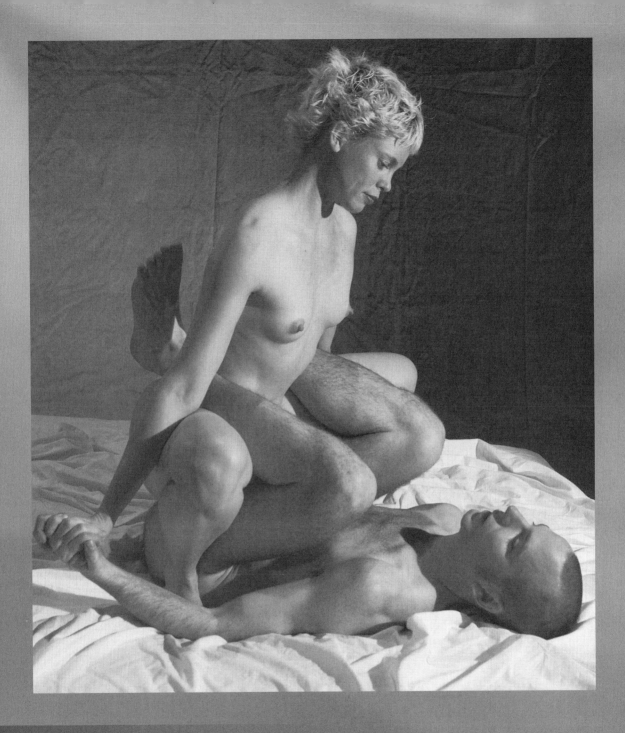

The pleasure of the pose: According to the original Kama

Sutra, this pose is "only apt for dangerous spirits and opened minds" since the "Amazon" is the woman who rides her man in the wildest and most primitive way. Here the woman is in charge.

The Trapeze

His Setup: Sit in a pseudo Prayer Squat Pose propped up on the edge of a bed or couch with knees apart. You'll want to be holding on to your lover's hips as the pose progresses.

Her Setup: Sit on top of your lover, straddling him as if in Seated Angle Pose. If possible bring the soles of your feet together. Now slowly drop your head back and arch your spine down toward the floor. You should feel as though you are upside-down in the hands of your lover.

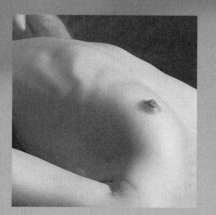
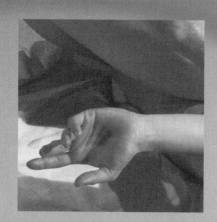
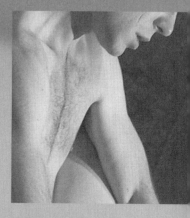

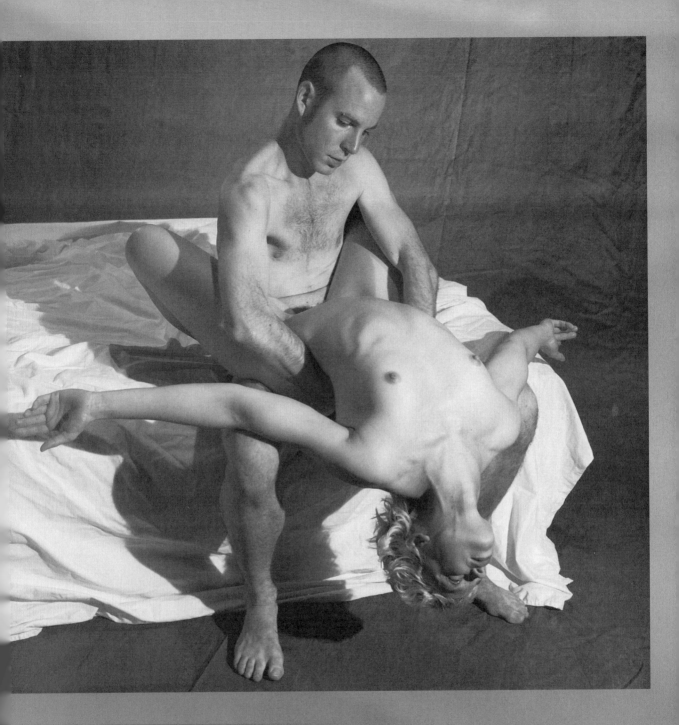

The pleasure of the pose: The man feels like a king in this position with his total view of his lover's body.

The Surprise

His Setup: Stand behind your lover, with your legs approximately one foot apart. Knees can be bent or straight. Press your body against your lover's butt and hug your arms around her waist.

Her Setup: Stand with your back to your lover and bend over at the waist. Relax your upper body in this forward bend position and simply breathe.

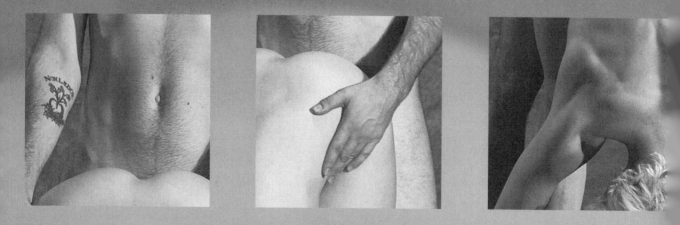

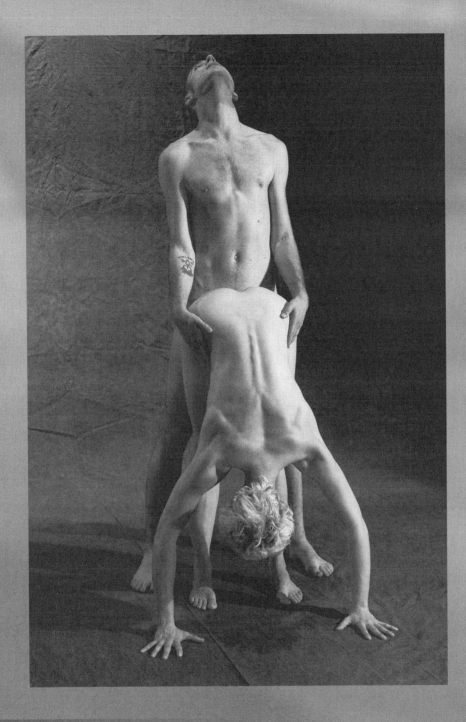

The pleasure of the pose: This position induces the
wildest and most primitive sex. The view from the man's perspective
includes two very erogenous zones—the anus and the butt. According to
the Kama Sutra, the male domination that the pose exerts and the total
relaxation in the woman makes for a brilliant surprise.

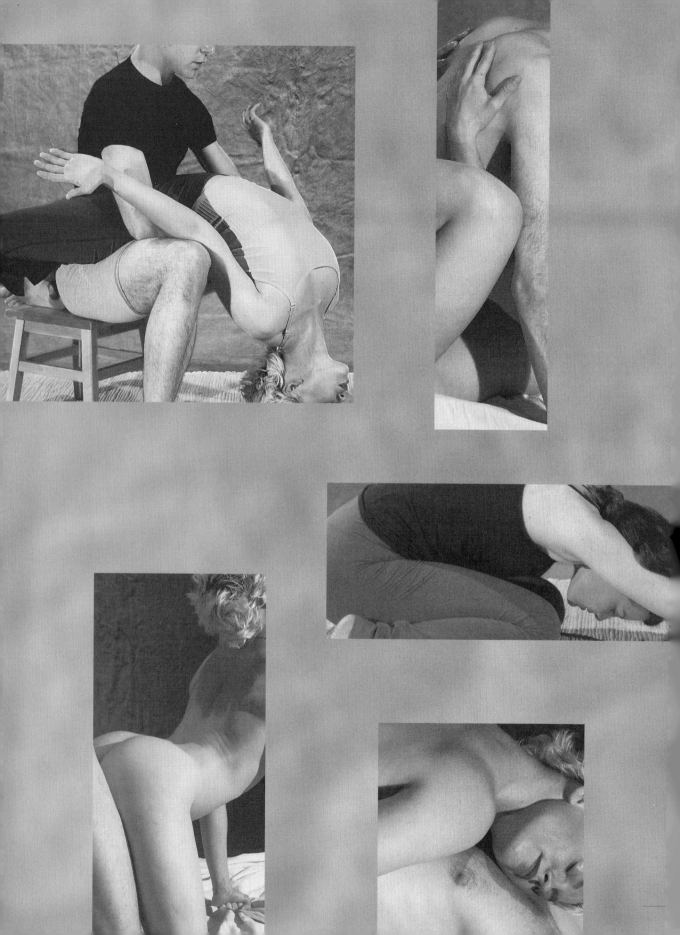

Index

Other Books by Ulysses Press

ASHTANGA YOGA FOR WOMEN: INVIGORATING MIND, BODY AND SPIRIT WITH POWER YOGA

Sally Griffyn, $17.95

Presents the exciting and empowering practice of power yoga in a balanced fashion that addresses the specific needs of female practitioners.

BALLET-FIT WORKOUT: DEVELOP STRENGTH, CONTROL, FLEXIBILITY & GRACE

Megan Connelly, Paula Baird-Colt & David McAllister, $16.95

Optimal health is the focus throughout *Ballet-Fit Workout*, and the authors show how classic dance training not only reshapes the body but also teaches mental focus and leads to a calm, refreshed mind.

THE LITTLE BIT NAUGHTY BOOK OF SEX

Dr. Jean Rogiere, $9.95

A handy pocket hardcover that is a fun, full-on guide to enjoying great sex.

THE LITTLE BIT NAUGHTY BOOK OF SEX POSITIONS

Siobhan Kelly, $9.95

Bored with the missionary position and in need of inspiration? Fully illustrated with 50 tastefully explicit color photos, *The Little Bit Naughty Book of Sex Positions* provides everything readers need to start using these thrilling new positions tonight.

NAUGHTY GIRLS' NIGHT IN

Shana Duthie & Stacey Jewell, $14.95

From enjoying a night of sexy fun with your girlfriends to starting a highly profitable home business, this book describes everything you need to know about in-home adult parties.

YOGA IN FOCUS: POSTURES, SEQUENCES AND MEDITATIONS

Jessie Chapman   photographs by Dhyan, $14.95

A beautiful celebration of yoga that's both useful for learning the techniques and inspiring in its artistic approach to presenting the body in yoga positions.

YOGA FOR PARTNERS: OVER 75 POSTURES TO DO TOGETHER

Jessie Chapman   photographs by Dhyan, $14.95

Features inspiring photos of the paired asanas. It teaches each partner how to synchronize their movements and breathing, bringing new lightness and enjoyment to any yoga practice.

To order these books call 800-377-2542 or 510-601-8301, fax 510-601-8307, e-mail ulysses@ulyssespress.com, or write to Ulysses Press, P.O. Box 3440, Berkeley, CA 94703. All retail orders are shipped free of charge. California residents must include sales tax. Allow two to three weeks for delivery.

ABOUT THE PHOTOGRAPHER

Andy Mogg is a well-known and much-published photographer. Born in England in 1954, he worked as a consultant, then writer and photographer. At seventeen he moved from London to Belgium, traveling and working his way through Europe, settling in the U.S. twenty years ago. He now runs a thriving photography studio in San Francisco. For more information, visit his website at www.dancingimages.com.

ABOUT THE MODELS

Sonya Smith dances professionally throughout the San Francisco Bay Area, creating and collaborating on aerial dance, site-specific dance,

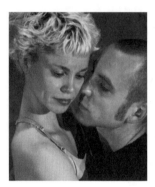 modern dance and improvisational performances. She is co-director and artist-in-residence of the renowned 848 Community Space in San Francisco.

Nol Simonse is a professional dancer and artist living in San Francisco.

ABOUT THE AUTHOR

Ellen Barrett, M.S., is known for her warm and intelligent approach to modern wellness. As a veteran CRUNCH™ instructor, renowned 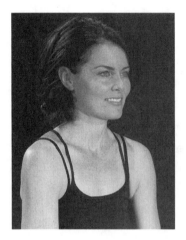 celebrity trainer and star of many international best-selling exercise videos, Ellen is one of the industry's most in-demand fitness personalities specializing in mind/body technique. "Yoga, meditation and other Eastern teachings can bring a great wealth of joy to humanity," she says, thus her career firmly entails helping people tune into their own inseparable mind and body. She currently splits her time between New York City and southern Connecticut, where she owns THE STUDIO, a yoga/Pilates fusion fitness center. For more information about Ellen, please visit her website at www.buffgirlfitness.com. *Sexy Yoga* is Ms. Barrett's first book.

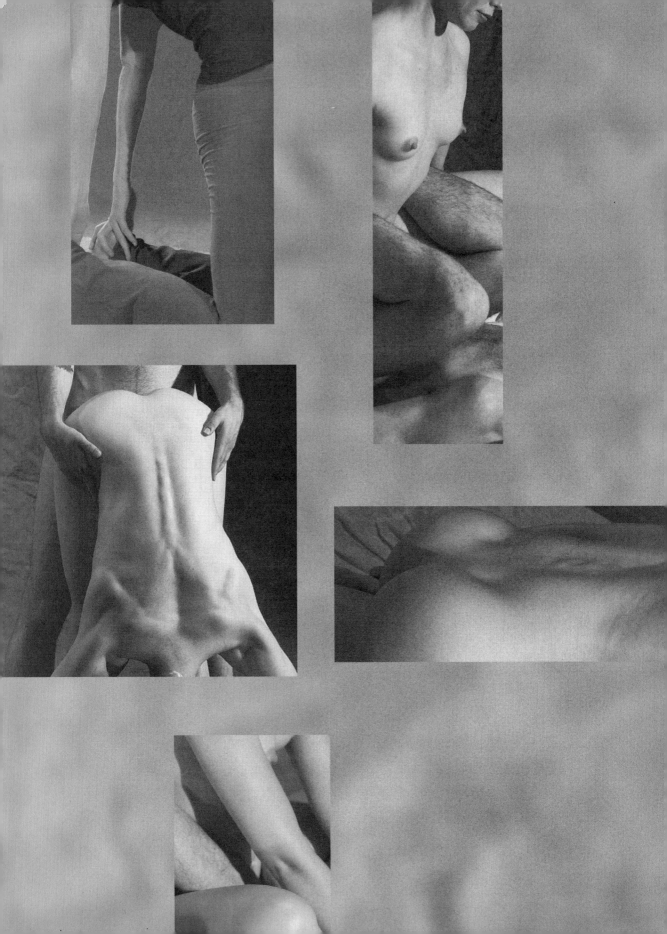